PRACTICAL FUELING FOR ENDURANCE ATHLETES

Your Nutrition Guide for Optimal Performance

Library of Congress Cataloging-in-Publication Data

Names: Van Horn, Kylee, 1986- author.
Title: Practical fueling for endurance athletes / Kylee Van Horn.
Description: Champaign, IL : Human Kinetics, 2026. | Includes
    bibliographical references and index.
Identifiers: LCCN 2024038946 (print) | LCCN 2024038947 (ebook) | ISBN
    9781718216785 (paperback) | ISBN 9781718216792 (epub) | ISBN
    9781718216808 (pdf)
Subjects: LCSH: Athletes--Nutrition. | Endurance sports--Training.
Classification: LCC TX361.A8 V36 2026 (print) | LCC TX361.A8 (ebook) |
    DDC 613.2--dc23/eng/20241029
LC record available at https://lccn.loc.gov/2024038946
LC ebook record available at https://lccn.loc.gov/2024038947

ISBN: 978-1-7182-1678-5 (print)

Copyright © 2026 by Flynutrition, LLC

This publication is written and published to provide accurate and authoritative information relevant to the subject matter presented. It is published and sold with the understanding that the author and publisher are not engaged in rendering legal, medical, or other professional services by reason of their authorship or publication of this work. If medical or other expert assistance is required, the services of a competent professional person should be sought.

The web addresses cited in this text were current as of August 2024, unless otherwise noted.

Senior Acquisitions Editor: Michelle Earle; **Developmental Editor:** Amy Stahl; **Copyeditor:** Erica Warren; **Proofreader:** Mary Elisabeth Frediani; **Indexer:** Rebecca L. McCorkle; **Permissions Manager:** Laurel Mitchell; **Graphic Designer:** Dawn Sills; **Cover Designer:** Keri Evans; **Cover Design Specialist:** Susan Rothermel Allen; **Photograph (cover):** Dan Patitucci / PatitucciPhoto; **Photographs (interior):** © Human Kinetics, unless otherwise noted; **Photo Asset Manager:** Laura Fitch; **Photo Production Manager:** Jason Allen; **Senior Art Manager:** Kelly Hendren; **Illustrations:** © Human Kinetics, unless otherwise noted; **Printer:** Versa Press

Human Kinetics books are available at special discounts for bulk purchase. Special editions or book excerpts can also be created to specification. For details, contact the Special Sales Manager at Human Kinetics.

Printed in the United States of America   10 9 8 7 6 5 4 3 2 1

The paper in this book is certified under a sustainable forestry program.

Human Kinetics   *United States and International*   *Canada*
1607 N. Market Street   Website: **US.HumanKinetics.com**   Website: **Canada.HumanKinetics.com**
Champaign, IL 61820   Email: info@hkusa.com   Email: info@hkcanada.com
USA   Phone: 1-800-747-4457

E8863

PRACTICAL FUELING FOR ENDURANCE ATHLETES

Your Nutrition Guide for Optimal Performance

Kylee Van Horn, LD, RDN

HUMAN KINETICS

CONTENTS

RECIPE FINDER

Chapter 10

FOREWORD

Why is endurance nutrition so complicated?

Between grams of carbohydrate per hour, adenosine triphosphate (ATP) production, sodium balance, and the Krebs cycle, it can feel like the simple act of fueling requires a dual PhD in chemistry and mathematics. Navigating diet culture's near-constant onslaught of misplaced messaging and wading through the bottomless pit of internet advice or ill-informed comments from other athletes can feel disheartening and overwhelming and can straight up make you feel crazy.

That's where Kylee and this book come in.

Even I, an elite athlete and journalist, find myself getting lost in the data and narratives about food and fueling that permeate our culture. Should I be taking more iron? Avoiding dairy? How the heck am I supposed to eat while running 100 miles?

Kylee has worked for years to demystify endurance fueling so athletes can tailor an approach that works for them and their individual needs. This book bridges the gap from her one-on-one practice working with some of the world's best endurance athletes, including runners who have had top finishes at the Western States Endurance Run and UTMB, so that everyday athletes can channel that information into sustainable action in their own practices.

Reading Kylee's advice is like having your own registered dietitian nutritionist in your pocket, helping you figure out what foods will fuel performance and what might be holding you back from breakthroughs. You won't find hard-to-follow meal plans or impossible recipes full of hard-to-find ingredients. There are no expensive supplements or intense protocols here—just good food and commonsense approaches made simple so that every athlete can step up to the starting line feeling confident, healthy, and well fueled.

She doesn't advocate for extreme approaches or cheap hacks. Kylee is an obsessive researcher, always digging into the data to see what works in the lab and then implementing it in her practice to identify what benefits athletes on the ground. Her writing simplifies even the most complex scientific ideas so that everyone can make better, more informed decisions about their diet and health when it comes to fueling for sport.

This book will help novice athletes and nutrition geeks alike fine-tune their fueling to reach their potential—no extreme diets or crazy supplements necessary.

The assertions in this book are backed by significant research and experience working with some of the world's best athletes. It also sends a radical message: Performance fueling isn't about what you weigh; it's about how well you fuel. Kylee's work stands above the rest by not focusing on weight in a world that's already all too obsessed with athletes' appearances.

If you want to step off the weight-loss treadmill and into breakthrough performances on the track, trail, court, field, or anywhere in between, this book will give you clear and actionable advice, supported with evidence and brief interviews to help you fuel your potential.

— Zoë Rom

PREFACE

I was 16 years old, standing in line to receive a T-shirt at a regional high school cross-country meet. What seemed like an insignificant interaction would become a profound memory of mine. I reached the front of the line, and those manning the table asked me what size T-shirt I wanted. I requested a small but received a medium. I asked again for a small shirt but was told they were saving those for the "smaller girls." Here I was, 5 feet 7 inches and 125 pounds, being told I didn't look like one of the smaller girls. Competitively running throughout high school and college, I was constantly faced with this ideal endurance runner image, always teetering between starving myself and overeating. My teammates in college were no different. I distinctly remember at least 25 percent of the team (male and female) having diagnosable eating disorders that were hidden or ignored. And the remainder of the team had to watch what we ate, which would be checked at the weekly weigh-ins in the training room. Apparently, to be the best, you had to look the best—the leanest, smallest version of yourself.

The idea that being thinner will make you faster pervades the world of endurance sports. It comes from all sides, including public opinion, medical professionals, coaches, trainers, and the media. The community instills this ideal into athletes at a young age, and it only continues as they grow. As a result, the longing for an ideal body chronically persists, pushing them to try the newest diet trends in hopes of discovering a performance advantage or achieving an endurance athlete image (whatever that is).

No one wants to address the obvious questions: What about the soul-crushing mental health challenges that come along with food and body obsession? What about the risks of injury and illness? What about the irreputable damage you are doing to your bones? What about the performance benefits you leave on the table when you try to manipulate your body by underfueling?

What if, instead, we were to flip the script and focus on fueling for performance to become a well-fed athlete, not a starving horse? I have experience working with thousands of endurance athletes, and without a doubt, being a healthy endurance athlete requires attention to the foundational nutrition skills, which have the biggest impact on health and performance first—things such as getting enough nutrition to match training volume and intensity, meeting micronutrient needs, timing nutrition correctly, hydrating properly, replenishing electrolytes, and developing a race fueling strategy. The problem with these skills is that they aren't sexy and won't get the most likes on social media.

Once you've built a strong nutritional foundation, then and only then should you focus on the minute details of your nutrition, the things that *might* give you a small advantage at best.

So, what have I found to be most effective for my athletes?

- Your daily nutrition strategy must fit *your* lifestyle, not someone else's.

- Learn to be adaptable. You should understand how to fuel on vacation, on work trips, when ordering at a restaurant, or when you are sick. The world will not end in these situations.

- Develop your race fueling strategy well in advance. Failing to practice is planning to fail. You put so much work into the training, so why not into your nutrition?

- Don't use supplements as a crutch. Doing so could backfire on you.

- Focus on rest and recovery tools just as much as your training.

As an endurance sports dietitian working in a world dominated by information overwhelm, I'm on a mission to separate facts from fads and set the record straight for endurance athletes who want to perform at their peak. This book is not the newest fad diet, an influencer cry for attention, or a walking advertisement for the hottest supplements. Its purpose is to provide you with a trusted resource that lays out the whats, whys, and hows of sports nutrition, no matter what endurance sport you compete in. It serves as a practical, science-based nutrition guide that's built around common challenges and questions from athletes I work with.

As you navigate the book, feel free to skip around to learn more about the things that interest you most. While it can be read cover to cover, it is designed to help you make immediate changes to your fueling strategy to help support both health and performance. The book is divided into two distinct parts: The first part helps you navigate the daily challenges of fueling yourself as an endurance athlete, while the second part supports you as you design, test, and implement a sport-specific race fueling strategy. Checklists, charts, and recipes are interspersed throughout to help you apply the nutrition information in a personalized way.

This book is meant to wade through all the ridiculous nutrition advice and gather the essential information into one sound reference to fuel all your endurance endeavors. Whether you are a beginner or advanced endurance athlete, I hope you will use this resource to properly fuel yourself to your next fastest time, to a race, or to whatever endurance project excites you. Remember: If you fuel it, you can do it.

ACKNOWLEDGMENTS

To my endurance hero in life and sport—my husband, Sean. Thanks for showing me what true grit and persistence looks like, for always challenging my views on the science and application of endurance sports nutrition, and for loving me through this thing we call life together.

To my right-hand training partner, wordsmith, comedian, and friend, Zoë.

To my dad, Tim, for nurturing my love of running and teaching me to uncover my talents in the sport.

To my forever cheer squad—my mom, Stacey; and my sister, Kameron.

To all the teammates, coaches, and friends I have made along the way, you have shaped me into the runner, coach, and sports dietitian who I am today. A special shout out to the late Tim Cook, my high school cross country and track coach, who passed away in a tragic car accident when I was a junior in high school. He made everyone feel like they were the most important runner out there and encouraged with kindness and led with humility. We could all use a little more of that in this world.

To those who have pushed themselves to their limits to achieve something beyond their wildest dreams. Hold tight to that feeling and use this book to guide you to many more achievements.

To all those who have been marginalized by the endurance community and wellness space. This book is for you. Long may you run, bike, swim, climb, row, and ski without uncertainty and fear of fueling. May you find this book refreshing, nonjudgemental and nonrestrictive in a way that allows for you to fuel for performance and nothing else.

And to all the endurance athletes out there (yes, all of you are an athlete), always remember: If you fuel it, you can do it.

PART I

ESSENTIALS OF ENDURANCE SPORTS NUTRITION

EATING TO TRAIN AND COMPETE

I would argue that no athlete ever has their nutrition plan 100 percent dialed in. There is always something we can improve on. That is what your focus should be when you are approaching the longer training sessions during your race-specific prep. In the off-season, you should devote time to trying to train the gut to handle higher calories, higher osmolality, more fluids. During race-specific prep, you should be focused on really dialing in your plan. Be willing to [make] mistakes by pushing too much in during your workouts to find out where that upper limit is for you. I'd much rather find that out in training than during a race. Finally, make sure you are working to find your specific needs for carbohydrates, electrolytes, and overall fluids per hour. Once you have those numbers sorted, you can start experimenting with what products and sources of the fuel work for you. Then you can start to figure out the logistics of getting your fuel on race day.

—Matt Hanson, professional triathlete and exercise scientist (personal communication, 2024)

To fuel himself to victory, Maurice Garin, the first winner of the Tour de France in 1903, reportedly ate at local pubs (Hurford, 2016), while Canadian runner Tom Longboat drank champagne during the 1908 Olympic marathon and unfortunately was not so lucky; he was forced to drop out at mile 19. Fueling tactics in the past included consuming alcohol and tea as well as eating everything from bananas to cake as a source of carbohydrates.

It wasn't really until 1965, when Gatorade first released its sports drink, that the importance of endurance-sports fueling really came into focus. Gatorade provided the means for an athlete to get calories, fluids, and sodium all from one source. It set the tone for what was to come in the sports nutrition world, where conventional wisdom is so saturated with both information and misinformation that it can be hard to discern the right way to fuel the body for performance.

Think of the most recent messaging you've heard or seen about sports nutrition. I'm going to guess that only about half of it was grounded in science or had practical applications to your life. While the baseline level of knowledge tends to vary in endurance-sports nutrition, you must focus on the foundational nutrition skills to fuel the body well and recover properly before homing in on the finer details.

I liken it to building a house. Without the proper foundation in place, the rest of the details don't matter because it will ultimately crumble. It's the same with your foundational nutrition skills. That's not to say that your foundation won't look different from another endurance athlete's foundation, but the skills must be in place. At the end of the day, nutrition must work for your lifestyle, and that's where the athlete disconnect often comes in. To put it more clearly, while there might be certain nutrition recommendations and practices for endurance athletes to follow, if you can't actually make the changes in a way that feels doable in the long term, then there is a disconnect between recommendations and reality. That gap between education and application is where this book becomes most useful. It provides a bridge and offers practical solutions to some of your toughest nutrition challenges.

Overwhelmed and confused, many endurance athletes struggle to wade through the ever-evolving world of sports nutrition to create a clear path forward. In a society where instant gratification is preferred, many athletes constantly waver between fad diets, the newest nutrition "hack," and dietary supplements to gain an extra advantage instead of actually investing time and resources into bettering their nutrition skills. Unfortunately, this can lead to a whole host of unintentional health and performance side effects, including hormonal imbalances, increased injury risk, decreased training adaptations, micronutrient deficiencies, and gut imbalances.

Endurance sports include a wide range of disciplines, intensities, and distances of activities, which can affect daily and intraworkout nutrition specifics and should not be presented as a one-size-fits-all recommendation. Because of the sheer amount of time and energy endurance athletes spend training and racing, their nutrition requires close attention to overall energy intake, since it can be all too easy to end up underfueled. And with high amounts of stress, micronutrients such as iron, calcium, and magnesium become even more important to include as part of an overall nutrition strategy. These micronutrients provide support for the body's endurance machine, allowing for proper energy production, muscle contraction, and structural support for bones and muscles. The intraworkout fuel plan must be approached like a puzzle with an intricate interplay of fluids, electrolytes, and calories all coming together to influence performance.

Most endurance athletes are not training for competition year-round and, therefore, go through different microcycles and macrocycles to periodize their training. A training microcycle is a shorter, more focused period that allows the body to be trained and overloaded. A training macrocycle is essentially your whole season with all the different periodized training components included. Similarly, nutrition can also be periodized to maximize training adaptations. On a micro level, nutrition can be adjusted daily to account for different training sessions. Macro-level nutrition can be adjusted based on the current part of the athlete's training cycle and on competition-specific goals.

Quite often, endurance athletes approach their nutrition haphazardly without a plan or any intention for what they're doing. They turn to supplements as a crutch to gain a performance edge, when what they really need to focus on is nutrition periodization and timing, hydration, and sleep before trying supplementation. That's what this book will help you sort out, with visuals such as the endurance-sports nutrition hierarchy of needs shown in figure 1.1. It stresses the importance of nutrition and lifestyle changes before introducing supplementation.

To prioritize this hierarchy appropriately, athletes must shift away from the hyped-up marketing of quick fixes and extreme methods and take a more rational approach to fueling that combines practicality and intention with intuition. Due to the busyness of everyday life and the push to keep doing more, more, more, many athletes have lost their innate ability to recognize and respond to hunger, fullness, and thirst cues. And while it is important to be able to fuel with intention to meet energy demands, our bodies are not calculated machines, and remembering that is also important for long-term physical and mental health.

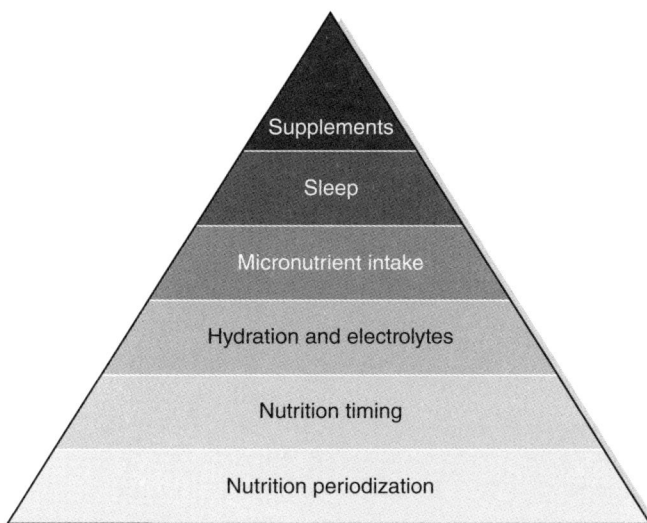

FIGURE 1.1 Endurance-sports nutrition hierarchy of foundational nutrition skills.

Calculating Energy Demands

When professional triathlete Matt Hanson started his career, he was training more than he ever had before during the summer months. However, he did not boost his caloric intake to help his body adapt to the increased training demands. For the first few years of his professional career, he struggled to perform at the Ironman World Championship every October. He thought that eating to hunger and drinking to thirst was good enough, despite weight falling off his frame. Rather than be concerned at the time, he thought it was a good thing to be "lighter and faster" on race day (Matt Hanson, personal communication, 2024).

Unfortunately, according to Hanson, this was a complete oversight on his part because while he was able to get through hard training sessions during the build, he didn't have the reserves necessary to compete at the intensities he wanted. He was unintentionally underfueling himself (Matt Hanson, personal communication, 2024). Fueling enough can be a tricky game for all endurance athletes. How do you know the right amount of food and fuel for your own endurance-sport endeavors? While there are many different opinions out there about the "right" amount, diet, or body composition, this book aims to take a different approach. This line of thinking is a more balanced, weight-neutral strategy that recognizes weight as *one factor among many* in performance, not the only factor.

Factors to Consider

It is important to recognize that messaging about weight and body composition is pervasive in endurance sports and can cause unnecessary long-term harm to you as an athlete. Performance nutrition is not the same as aesthetic nutrition—keep in mind, this is not a bodybuilding book. Sport and body stereotypes can lead coaches, parents, and athletes to oversimplify and believe they need to look a certain way to perform at a certain level. We can't deny that weight is one factor that *may* play a role in endurance-sports performance, but we know that how an athlete performs involves much more than weight and body composition.

Ron Thompson, PhD, FAED, CEDS, came up with a list of 40 factors from sports psychology research that play a role in sports performance (see table 1.1). Taking the time to recognize and respect all of them can turn our attention and conversations away from weight (Rapp et al. 2021).

By switching your thought process from "What more can I do to restrict and lose weight?" to a more productive mindset of "What factors am I not focusing on by focusing on weight?" you can have a more well-rounded view of ways to improve performance.

TABLE 1.1   **Factors That Play a Role in Sports Performance**

Genetics	Training	Practice	Coaching
Physical health	Balance	Body composition	Coordination
Courage	Endurance	Nutrition	Quickness
Reaction time	Rest	Sleep	Speed
Strength	$\dot{V}O_2$max	Weight	Mental health
Mental preparation	Mental toughness	Anticipation	Coachability
Competitiveness	Commitment	Concentration	Confidence
Desire	"Heart"	Intelligence	Motivation
Perfectionism	"Playing with pain"	Poise	Teammate dynamic
Respect	Sacrifice	Teamwork	Hard work

Courtesy of Ron Thompson, PhD, FAED, and Roberta Sherman, PhD.

Energy Requirements

Simply put, a calorie is a unit of energy that the body uses to power its systems. Consuming an adequate number of calories is essential for any endurance athlete who is training and racing. Without sufficient calories, athletes struggle to adapt to training stressors and have a higher risk of injury and illness.

There are four macronutrients that contain calories: alcohols, proteins, carbohydrates, and fats. Energy demands vary depending on an athlete's body frame size, genetics, training load, and intensity. The mix of macronutrients an athlete should consume depends on training and competitive needs and goals. Understanding how your body uses each macronutrient can help you determine your body's unique needs.

Proteins

Proteins have thousands of uses in the body, including broader functions such as muscle and cell repair, immune support, enzyme production, and neurotransmitter production. Endurance athletes put their bodies under a lot of physical and mental stress during training and competition. With adequate protein intake, muscles adapt and strengthen under stressors, enzymes are produced to help with energy production, and the body fortifies the immune system to shield against illness. Low protein intake can lead to fatigue, poor recovery times, immune system suppression, and increased risk of muscle and tendon injuries.

In terms of energy, protein contains four calories per gram. When proteins are taken in, they travel to the stomach, where stomach acid breaks them down into shorter strands and some amino acids. This process continues in the small intestine, until the proteins are broken into individual amino acids, which are then absorbed and delivered to the appropriate areas in the body.

Your body needs 20 different amino acids to function properly, as shown in table 1.2. It can produce 11 of them internally; these are called *nonessential* or *conditionally essential amino acids*, and most of them can be found in foods such as nuts, seeds, grains, and vegetables. The remaining 9 are called *essential amino acids*, which cannot be produced internally and must be taken in from foods such as soy, quinoa, animal products, and dairy. Table 1.3, while not fully comprehensive, provides a quick reference for some of the most common foods containing certain amino acids.

TABLE 1.2   Essential, Nonessential, and Conditionally Essential Amino Acids

Essential	Nonessential	Conditionally essential
Histidine	Alanine	Arginine
Isoleucine	Asparagine	Cysteine
Leucine	Aspartate	Glutamine
Lysine	Glutamate	Glycine
Methionine	Serine	Proline
Phenylalanine		Tyrosine
Threonine		
Tryptophan		
Valine		

Some foods contain all 20 amino acids and are considered complete sources of protein, while others are incomplete. You do not need to eat complementary protein-containing foods together at the same time to get all 20 amino acids. As long as you consume a variety of protein-containing foods throughout the day, your body will put them together.

Out of all the amino acids, those that are most critical for endurance athletes are the three branched-chain amino acids (BCAAs): leucine, isoleucine, and valine. Aptly named for their chemical structure, BCAAs provide endurance athletes with the highest rate of muscle protein synthesis. Hello, muscle recovery and decreased soreness! BCAAs have also been shown to play an important role in cell signaling, glucose and fat metabolism, and gut integrity.

It is important for endurance athletes to have some awareness of protein-containing foods and how much protein those foods contain. Table 1.4, while not fully comprehensive, provides a quick reference for some of the most common high-protein foods and the corresponding amount of protein in those foods.

TABLE 1.3   Best Foods to Consume for Specific Amino Acids

Histidine	Beef, pork chops, tuna, tofu, milk, eggs
Isoleucine	Beef, chicken, tofu, milk, lentils, peas
Leucine	Chicken, beef, tofu, pumpkin seeds, yogurt
Lysine	Beef, chicken, eggs, tofu, cheese
Methionine	Pork chops, crab, Brazil nuts, turkey
Phenylalanine	Dairy products, nuts, seeds, tofu
Threonine	Carrots, bananas, edamame, eggs
Tryptophan	Turkey, pineapple, tofu, eggs, seeds
Valine	Tempeh, beef, eggs, yogurt
Alanine	Chicken, turkey, beans, edamame
Asparagine	Potatoes, beef, eggs, nuts
Aspartate	Asparagus, eggs, lentils, avocados, oysters
Glutamate	Cheese, tomatoes, nuts, mushrooms
Serine	Walnuts, lentils, chickpeas, eggs
Arginine	Black beans, chickpeas, pumpkin seeds
Cysteine	Cottage cheese, chicken, beef, yogurt
Glutamine	Red cabbage, eggs, milk, red kidney beans
Glycine	Turkey, chicken, peanuts, quinoa, eggs
Proline	Cheese, tofu, gelatin, casein protein powder
Tyrosine	Sesame seeds, cheese, fish, nuts, beef, pork, lamb, chicken, turkey

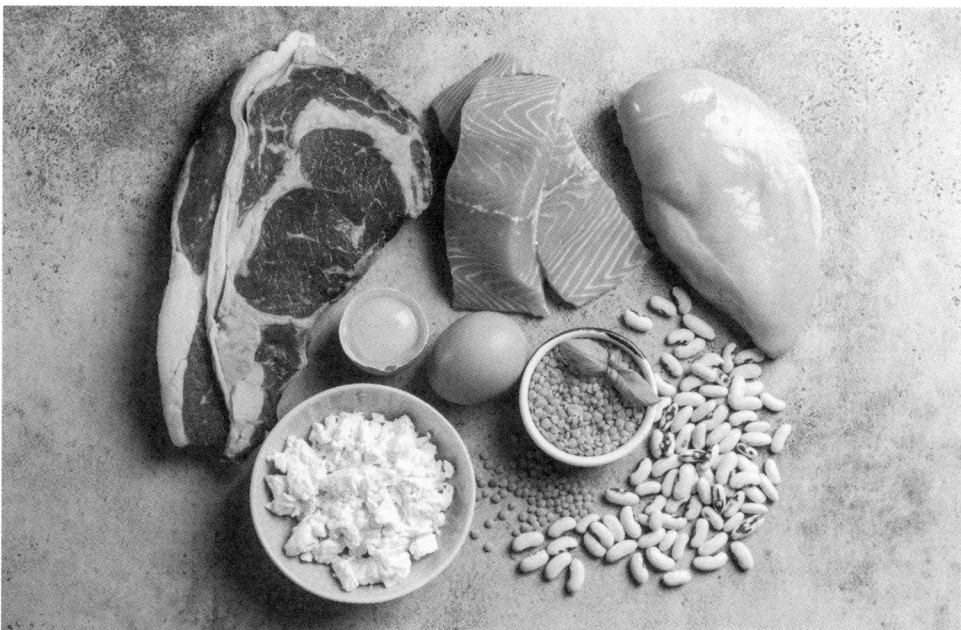

Elena Yeryomenko/500px Plus/Getty Images

Meats, dairy, eggs, beans, and fish are all key sources of amino acids.

TABLE 1.4 Food Containing High Amounts of Protein

Type of food	Amount of food	Protein content
Chia seeds	2 tbsp	4 g
Egg	1 small	6 g
Chickpeas	1/2 cup (115 g)	6 g
Cashews	1/4 cup (35 g)	6 g
Black beans	1/2 cup (115 g)	7 g
Cheddar cheese	1 oz (30 g)	7 g
Soy milk	8 oz (240 mL)	7 g
Quinoa	1 cup (230 g) cooked	8 g
2% milk	8 oz (240 mL)	8 g
Peanut butter	2 tbsp	8 g
Greek yogurt	1 cup (230 g)	14 g
Tofu	4 oz (115 g)	14 g
2% cottage cheese	1 cup (230 g)	23 g
Tempeh	4 oz (115 g)	23 g
Seitan	4 oz (115 g)	24 g
Shrimp	4 oz (115 g)	27 g
Salmon filet	4 oz (115 g)	29 g
Ground beef	4 oz (115 g)	29 g
Pork chop	4 oz (115 g)	33 g
Chicken breast	4 oz (115 g)	35 g

Carbohydrates

Carbohydrates are the primary source of energy production for endurance athletes. Coming in at four calories per gram, carbohydrates are used in the mitochondria to help power the body. When consumed, carbohydrates are broken down into glucose and then either used for energy production or stored in the muscles or liver as glycogen, which can be used for energy production during exercise.

Carbohydrates are typically categorized into three types found in our food: sugar, starch, and fiber. From there, depending on their chemical structure, foods can be categorized as simple or complex. Simple carbohydrates (sugars) are straight-chain carbon molecules that are easily broken down and cause a quick rise and drop in blood sugar, while complex carbohydrates (starch or fiber) are branched-chain carbon molecules that are slowly broken down and cause a gradual rise and drop in blood sugar.

It is unhelpful for endurance athletes to classify simple versus complex carbohydrates as bad versus good. A better frame is for endurance athletes to consider using simple and complex carbohydrates strategically based on workout timing and training load. A quick, simple carbohydrate source can be beneficial for athletes to have before a workout to get an initial energy boost and preserve glycogen stores. After exercise, simple carbohydrates provide a quick and easy way to replace glycogen stores. On heavier training days when appetite may be suppressed and carbohydrate needs are higher, simple carbohydrates can meet nutritional needs without making you feel overly stuffed. One to two hours outside of the postworkout window, complex carbohydrates may be preferred because they promote satiety, provide extra vitamins and minerals, and keep blood sugar more stable. Table 1.5 provides an easy reference for carbohydrate types.

TABLE 1.5 Simple Versus Complex Carbohydrate-Containing Foods

Simple carbohydrates	Complex carbohydrates
Maple syrup	Brown rice
Honey	Oats
White pasta	Quinoa
White bread	Potatoes (white and sweet)
White rice	Wheat
Milk	Barley
Milk products	Beans
Raw sugar	Lentils
Fruit juice	Peas
	Bulgur

Fats

No, eating fats doesn't cause you to get fat. However, fats are the most concentrated energy source in the body. With nine calories per gram, they contain more than twice the amount of energy than their carbohydrate and protein counterparts. And although they are energy dense, fats are digested more slowly for energy production than carbohydrates.

Fats play several roles in the body:

- Absorption of fat-soluble vitamins (vitamins A, D, E, and K)
- Building blocks of hormones, particularly estrogen and testosterone
- Component of the lipid bilayer in cells, which is particularly important for endurance athletes who have high rates of cell breakdown due to training stressors
- Insulation and protection of organs
- Support of hair, skin, and nail health
- Signaling and transport for various cellular and physiological processes
- Nerve function

Athletes who limit fat consumption to less than 20 percent of total calorie consumption may be putting themselves at risk for fat-soluble vitamin deficiencies, hormonal imbalances, and hair, skin, and nail issues. Severely limiting fat intake should only occur during a carbohydrate increase or before a race to avoid gastrointestinal distress.

There are three main categories of fatty acids: polyunsaturated, monounsaturated, and saturated. Saturated fatty acids are solid at room temperature and are named for their carbon structure, which is surrounded, or saturated, by hydrogen atoms. Monounsaturated and polyunsaturated fatty acids are liquid at room temperature and contain hydrogen atoms but are not surrounded by them, and both have a positive effect on the cardiorespiratory system. Refer to table 1.6 for examples of different types of fats.

TABLE 1.6   Types and Sources of Fats

Saturated	Monounsaturated	Polyunsaturated
Red meats	Olive oil	Fish
Poultry	Canola oil	Fish oil
Dairy products	Peanut oil	Chia seeds
Lard	Sesame oil	Flax seeds
Coconut oil	Avocado	Hemp seeds
Palm oil	Almonds	Walnuts
Cocoa butter	Peanuts	Algal oil
Processed foods	Cashews	Pine nuts
	Pumpkin seeds	Sunflower seeds
	Sesame seeds	
	Olives	

How Do We Make All Our Energy?

We all have the ability to make energy from the foods we eat, as well as produce it from stored energy sources to power all the body's systems. Endurance athletes use three main energy systems to support performance during exercise: phosphagen, anaerobic glycolysis, and aerobic metabolism. Athletes rely on both fat and carbohydrate metabolism to sustain energy production; however, the intensity and duration of exercise will determine the proportion of fats versus carbohydrates used to maintain energy supplies.

• *The phosphagen system* is reserved mainly for short bursts of quick energy. It uses some ATP and some stored creatine phosphate to produce energy. ATP carries molecules that fuel basic physiological functions throughout the body. The phosphagen system produces enough energy for bursts of activity lasting up to 10 seconds, but after that point, the body relies on other systems that use fats, carbohydrates, and proteins to help keep the energy production going.

• *Anaerobic glycolysis* is the process by which the body breaks down glucose or glycogen (stored carbohydrate) to help make ATP when oxygen is low. One molecule of glucose can produce two units of ATP for energy production using this system. This process is mostly useful during high-intensity exercise and can serve as one of the main sources of fuel during exercise that lasts one to two minutes. It is important to note that carbohydrates are the only macronutrients that can be used to produce ATP without oxygen readily available in the system.

• *Aerobic metabolism* plays a dominant role in energy production for most endurance athletes who participate in longer events. This process involves a series of energy-producing steps (three parts: glycolysis, Krebs cycle, and oxidative phosphorylation) in the mitochondria, with oxygen present, to produce a constant supply of ATP. Both carbohydrates and fats are used to produce energy.

For every molecule of glucose that undergoes aerobic metabolism, 36 units of ATP are produced. Endurance athletes must understand that exogenous consumption of carbohydrates (carbohydrates consumed from fuel sources, not made internally) is required to keep the aerobic energy production process going. To fuel at rest without exogenous carbohydrates, the body stores carbohydrates mainly in the liver and muscles, with a tiny amount stored in brain, heart, and kidney cells. When in need of energy, the body uses glycogen stores by way of glycogenolysis. Whole-body glycogen stores are around 600 grams total, which is about 2,400 calories worth of energy that the body can use during exercise (Robinson 2010). Once these glycogen stores are depleted, the body relies on exogenous carbohydrates, fats, and broken-down proteins for energy production. Without carbohydrates, it can be hard to continue going at a higher percentage of maximal oxygen consumption ($\dot{V}O_2$max); if you don't take in carbohydrates, you may have to slow down.

While fats are always being used for energy production, when exercising at lower intensities for longer periods of time (between 25 and 70 percent $\dot{V}O_2$max), reliance on fats to produce energy becomes more important (Baker, McCormick, and Robergs 2010). Lipolysis involves breaking down stored fat into glycerol and free fatty acids, which are transported to the mitochondria, where they produce ATP. This process takes place much more slowly than the Krebs cycle but also yields a high amount of energy.

The Role of $\dot{V}O_2$max

Put simply, $\dot{V}O_2$max is the maximum rate of oxygen use during exercise. Often used as a marker for fitness, higher $\dot{V}O_2$max *usually but not always* relates to better fitness levels. The more oxygen you can bring to working muscles, the more energy you can produce. Think of it like your car's gas mileage. The higher your $\dot{V}O_2$max, the better performance you can get out of each breath. While $\dot{V}O_2$max can be trained to some extent, many factors affect it, including sex, genetics, age, and altitude.

So what does this have to do with nutrition? It's critical to understand that at different intensities of exercise, your body is using different percentages of fats *and* carbohydrates. Read that again. Your body is ideally always using both fats and carbohydrates at the same time for energy production, but at different percentages.

Fats are the predominant source of energy production for less than 40 percent $\dot{V}O_2$max, while they make up about half of energy production at 45 to 65 percent of one's $\dot{V}O_2$max. Above 65 percent $\dot{V}O_2$max, carbohydrates start to dominate in energy production. The point where an athlete goes from using fats to using carbohydrates is called the *crossover point*. The more aerobically trained an individual is, the more efficient they will be at using fats.

It can be helpful to think of using carbohydrates and fats and building your fueling plan not as one versus the other but rather, depending on goals, as what makes the most sense for energy production. For instance, for short, quick bursts of exercise—sprinting, going uphill, or doing quick moves like in an obstacle course race—you are likely using more anaerobic pathways for energy production, which requires mostly carbohydrates. As intensity decreases and duration increases, like in a marathon and beyond, you start to use a mix of anaerobic and aerobic systems, increasing the percentage of fats you use and changing up your fueling plan requirements.

Endurance-Sports Nutrition Periodization

Depending on your sport, your goals, and whether it's race season or off-season, nutrition needs can and will change. Periodized nutrition can be defined as combining training with nutrition or using nutrition alone to aid in obtaining adaptations that support exercise performance. In the literature, the term *periodized nutrition* is not well defined or understood. Most athletes focus on acute recovery and fueling strategies, but not necessarily on long-term outcomes, through dietary manipulation. For the purposes of this book, periodized nutrition is the change in nutrition in response to different periods of training, which could happen on a macro-, meso-, or microcycle scale.

While different nutritional periodization methods could be used to achieve different goals, this book will explain how to change up nutrition on a micro scale (daily) basis as well as a meso scale (i.e., preseason, race block, off-season). Within these cycles, macronutrients—proteins, carbohydrates, and fats—will vary in daily amounts depending on the individual's intended goals.

But What About the Low-Carb, High-Fat (LCHF) Diet?

No matter what body type you have, your body has stored an abundance of fatty acids. Ultra-endurance events are typically completed at a lower percentage of $\dot{V}O_2$max and done at a much slower pace than their marathon counterparts. Theoretically, it makes sense for some ultra-endurance-focused athletes to want to tap into fat stores for energy production for these events. Proponents of this strategy recommend it to reduce stress on the gastrointestinal system during training and racing, decrease inflammation (self-reported), and increase recovery times.

The outcomes of a LCHF dietary strategy include becoming more fat-adapted, being more efficient at using fats as fuel, and achieving maximum fat oxidation rates (i.e., using more fats at a higher percentage of $\dot{V}O_2$max). The main concept of a LCHF diet is that an athlete's diet will consist of more than 70 percent fats and 2 to 5 percent carbohydrates per day. Carbohydrates are used strategically around key workouts and long runs. Because you are consuming a higher amount of fats overall, you can adapt to the changes in diet in as little as 10 days; however, it typically takes a month.

So, what are the downsides? Unfortunately, if something sounds too good to be true, it usually is. This is not an overall winning solution for endurance athletes. There are some potential problems with this way of fueling that you'll need to consider before jumping in.

1. *Inability to train at higher percentages of $\dot{V}O_2$max:* This can limit an athlete's development because carbohydrates are necessary to perform and adapt when doing high-intensity intervals targeted at improving $\dot{V}O_2$max.

2. *Downregulation of carbohydrate utilization:* Using a higher percentage of fats versus carbohydrates in your daily diet and in training can downregulate the body's ability to use carbohydrates efficiently. Reducing carbohydrate consumption can decrease the number of glucose transporters in the small intestine, which can increase the risk of gastrointestinal distress. Ideally, you are always consuming some amount of carbohydrates during exercise to keep it running smoothly. Without any exogenous carbohydrate intake during exercise, the body will struggle to keep moving efficiently, and your pace will be forced to slow.

3. *Increased risk of bone stress injuries:* Having fewer carbohydrates coming into the body can increase levels of CTX (a marker of bone breakdown) and decrease levels of P1NP (a marker of bone building). Even under conditions of high energy availability but low carbohydrate availability, reduced bone-formation markers has been observed (Fensham et al. 2022).

At this time, the LCHF diet does not seem to produce any significant performance benefits when compared to a higher carbohydrate diet. Seemingly, what could be more beneficial is matching carbohydrate intake to exercise duration and intensity, which is the foundation of sports nutrition periodization.

Combined recommendations from the American College of Sports Medicine (ACSM) and the International Society of Sports Nutrition (ISSN) for macronutrient needs for endurance athletes are as follows:

Protein: 1.6 to 2.5 grams per kilogram of body weight per day

Carbohydrate: 3 to 12 grams per kilogram of body weight per day

Fat: 0.8 to 2.0 grams per kilogram of body weight per day

To use the nutrition periodization model and meet energy requirements, endurance athletes can put a system in place to define what and how much to eat on different types of training days. The athlete's plate model, shown in figure 1.2, is an easy-to-understand system that tends to be a more sustainable method for endurance athletes to include periodized nutrition in their routine. This framework was developed as a nutrition education tool to define how meal composition would ideally look depending on training load (volume × intensity).

The athlete's plate model includes a definition for each type of training day—easy, moderate, hard, and extra hard—which I created specifically for endurance athletes and their macronutrient needs. It allows an endurance athlete to use the different classifications to determine how much fuel they need for that day. The type of training is defined as follows:

- *Easy day:* Rest day; up to 60 minutes of easy-effort training.
- *Moderate day:* 61 minutes to 2 hours of easy-effort training or up to 60 minutes of high-intensity interval training (HIIT).
- *Hard day:* 2 to 3 hours of easy-effort training or 61 to 120 minutes of HIIT.
- *Extra hard day:* Beyond 3 hours of training. There is no defined visual plate as exercise duration increases; however, that does not mean that intake should not increase. Many endurance athletes I work with need a higher category of intake due to increased training volume, and an extra hard day fits the bill.

Once you know the basic framework, you can apply the combined ACSM and ISSN recommendations for endurance athletes to estimate nutritional needs and use it as a periodized model to support training and performance goals, as shown in table 1.7.

TABLE 1.7   Macronutrient Needs Based on Type of Training Day

Type of training day	Protein	Carbohydrate	Fat
Easy	1.6 g/kg body weight	3 g/kg body weight	0.8 g/kg body weight
Moderate	1.8 g/kg body weight	5 g/kg body weight	1.0 g/kg body weight
Hard	2.0 g/kg body weight	7 g/kg body weight	1.2 g/kg body weight
Extra hard	2.2 g/kg body weight	9 g/kg body weight	1.4 g/kg body weight

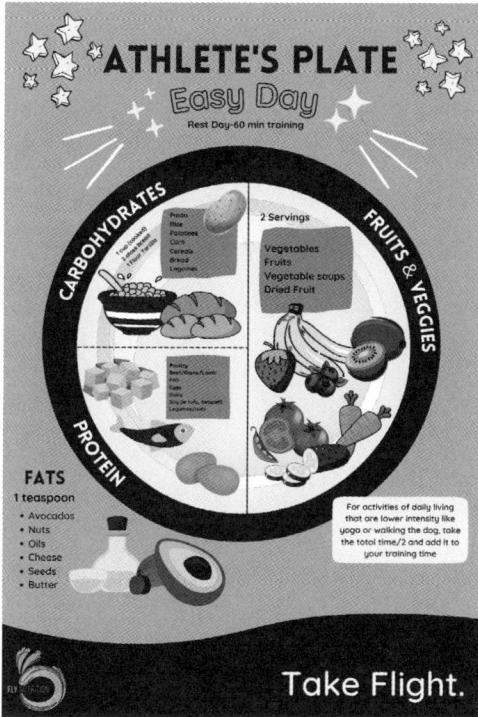

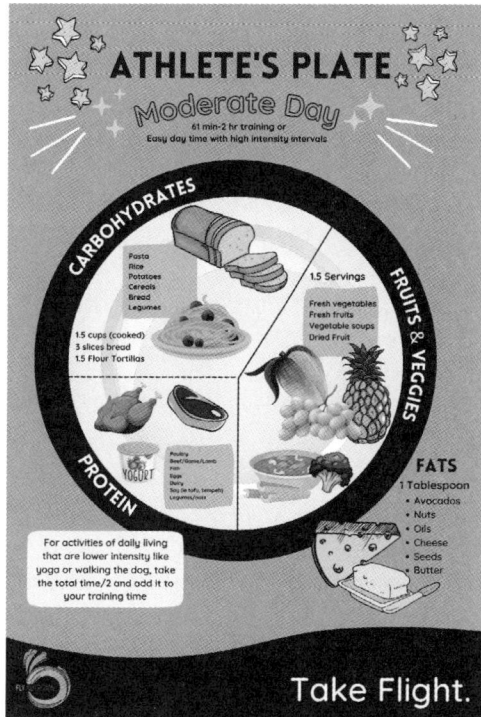

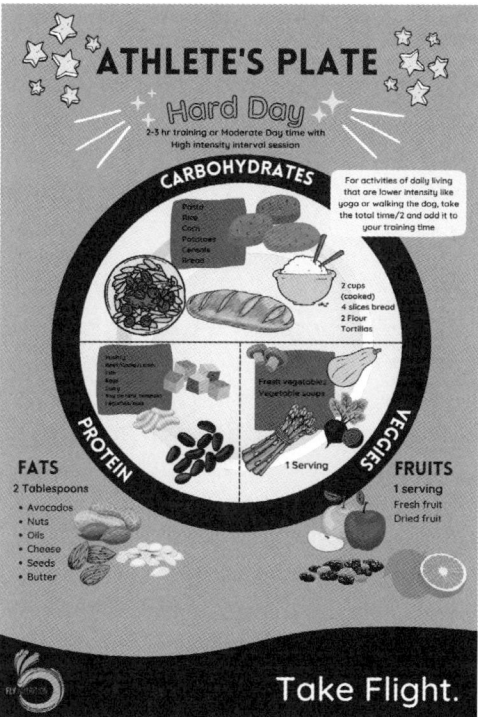

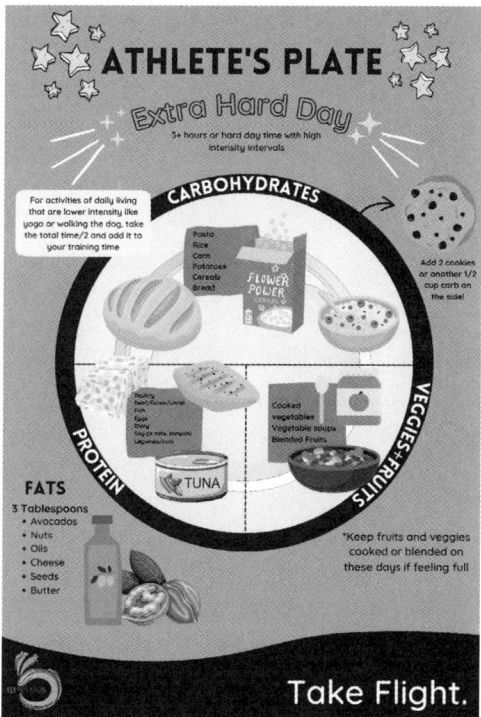

FIGURE 1.2 Athlete's plate models: Easy day, moderate day, hard day, and extra hard day.

Keep in mind that this framework is formulated based on a continuum, so if you engage in more training, your macronutrient needs increase. It also does not exist as a hard-and-fast framework and should be used in conjunction with hunger and fullness recognition to fuel properly overall.

What About Calories and Tracking Nutrition?

Endurance athletes tend to have a complicated relationship with tracking their overall calorie intake. Many have been taught to count calories as a means of weight control, forcing them into a void of restriction and obsession that can lead down a path of disordered eating. Others may track their intake to determine whether they are getting enough overall nutrition to support their training and performance goals. And while, yes, calories are an important piece of the energy requirement equation, counting calories and tracking food intake long-term can be time-consuming, obsessive, and unsustainable.

On the flip side, for a certain portion of the endurance-athlete population, temporary tracking of intake can provide some clarity about holes in the diet from a macro- or micronutrient perspective. For those who want to gain such awareness, using an app-based tracking system such as Cronometer or MyFitnessPal can give you a better idea of your overall energy intake and specific micronutrient intakes. Keep in mind these are still just estimates. Tracking apps have no idea what your metabolism, stress levels, or postexercise oxygen consumption rates are. It is well known that humans tend to significantly underestimate their total energy intake, which can affect the accuracy of tracking system results (Murakami and Livingstone 2015). Add in the confounding variable that wearable fitness tracking devices across all brands are inaccurate to some degree, and you've got an imperfect tool for estimation (Fuller et al. 2020). The only way to truly know your macro- and micronutrient requirements is to be hooked up to a metabolic device around the clock. That's unrealistic, right?

This is precisely why it's important for endurance athletes to hold food tracking metrics lightly while gaining awareness around intake. Numbers can be helpful to some extent, but it's important to have a system that works most of the time and can be adapted in different situations. The athlete's plate model can be an effective framework to help you understand your intake needs, but it's still just a tool. Without tuning in to your body's hunger and fullness cues, you are still just treating your body like a machine, not a human.

Hunger, Fullness, and the Psychological Side of Eating

When fueling yourself properly as an endurance athlete, you must recognize there are many reasons for eating. Food can function as fuel, but it is also so much more than that. It can hold memories and emotions, and it is meant to be enjoyed. This is also why it is important to not treat your body as a machine and obsess about numbers and metrics. When you focus solely on numbers, you may lose sight of your actual body signals for hunger and fullness, not to mention that eating becomes more of a chore than it used to be.

Through a scientific lens, hunger is a signal from the body reminding us that we should consume fuel. Hunger is influenced by many factors, and everyone experiences different levels and types of hunger responses. Hunger and fullness are regulated by a complex system of hormonal and neural signals. Big players in this equation are leptin, ghrelin, and peptide YY. Leptin and peptide YY both signal to the body that it is satisfied and doesn't need more nutrition, while ghrelin indicates to the body that it needs more fuel. Alterations or abnormalities in these hormones can cause the body to become dysregulated concerning hunger and fullness recognition and response.

Hunger recognition usually starts with being able to identify symptoms of hunger such as shakiness, low energy, a growling stomach, brain fog, and problems focusing. You may find it helpful to use a hunger and fullness scale. This rating system can help you gain more awareness of your own body's signals and recognize and respond appropriately to hunger and fullness cues. The rating system was popularized in 1995 by Evelyn Tribole and Elyse Resch when they introduced the scale in their book *Intuitive Eating: A Revolutionary Program That Works* and has since promoted a more mindful and body respectful approach to fueling (see figure 1.3).

Using this scale, you ideally want to fall between a five and a seven rating, which indicates satisfaction in the current moment. The better you get at recognizing and responding appropriately to hunger and fullness signals from your body, the less likely you are to under- or overfuel.

1. **Ravenous:** Physically ill and nauseated.

2. **Extremely hungry:** Moody, I have a headache, and I feel empty.

3. **Hungry:** Stomach is growling, and I need energy.

4. **"I could eat something.":** Stomach is slightly empty.

5. **Neutral:** No thoughts of food or signals from the body.

6. **Mildly full:** Full and satisfied.

7. **Satisfied:** Full but not uncomfortable unless I eat any more.

8. **Uncomfortably full:** A little bit overfull.

9. **Stuffed:** Like I overate on Thanksgiving.

10. **Binged full:** Physically sick.

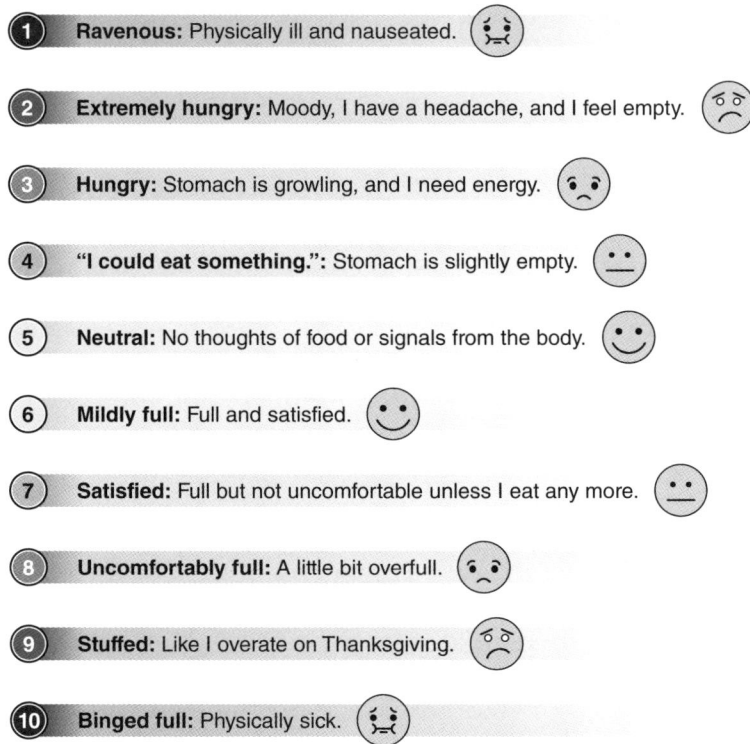

FIGURE 1.3   Hunger and fullness rating scale for endurance athletes.

Adapted from Tribole and Resch (1995).

The following are additional ways to best gauge whether you are hungry and recognize when you are full enough:

1. Take a moment to pause throughout your day and ask yourself if you are hungry.
2. Eat slowly and do a body scan to recognize how your body feels and to see if you are satisfied or full. This can be particularly difficult if you are distracted during meals and snacks.
3. Do body scans periodically to evaluate your mood and assess whether you are truly hungry or if you are feeling some other emotion.

While endurance athletes should be aware of their recognition and response patterns toward hunger and fullness, there are a few problems with simply paying attention to these signals as the core of fueling and nutrition. Endurance exercise can decrease appetite by increasing peptide YY and leptin levels but decreasing ghrelin levels (Douglas et al. 2015).

Hunger exists in many forms, and not all of them require you to eat to satisfy them.

- *Biological hunger* is the type of hunger mentioned previously that indicates its presence with physical symptoms.

- *Emotional hunger* is a response to emotions such as joy, sadness, anger, and stress. For some athletes, fueling is an automatic response to feeling emotions. In these situations, it is important to gain awareness of your emotions and have a toolbox of responses instead of automatically resorting to eating. In many cases of emotional eating, working with a licensed mental health professional can be beneficial to get past using food as a coping mechanism.

- *Habitual hunger* is a complex type of hunger that causes you to eat out of habit rather than actual hunger. In certain situations, this may be beneficial. For instance, if you get in the habit of eating breakfast between seven a.m. and nine a.m., that can be helpful if you tend to forget to eat because you are busy with work. However, fueling constantly with paired situations throughout the day can make it difficult to fuel intentionally and can cause you to lose sight of actual hunger and fullness cues.

- *Practical hunger* is important to mention for endurance athletes because the duration and intensity of endurance exercise, along with weather conditions (e.g., heat), can decrease appetite overall. This is why it is common for an endurance athlete to lose their appetite after a longer bout of training (more than 90 minutes). Practical hunger means you recognize that your training requires you to fuel yourself despite the loss of appetite. For instance, having an energy-dense smoothie after a workout could be an appropriate response to practical hunger.

What Happens If You Don't Fuel Enough?

Fueling properly as an endurance athlete can be a challenge, especially if you don't know how much is enough for your body. You also have to figure out how to match your training volume and intensity to your eating.

In 2014, the International Olympic Committee (IOC) came out with a consensus statement that addressed what can happen if athletes don't fuel enough to match their training demands (Mountjoy et al. 2023). Relative energy deficiency in sport (RED-S) is the overarching term used to describe athletes who experience the signs and symptoms of low energy availability (LEA). LEA is defined as a mismatch between an athlete's energy intake and energy expenditure, which leaves the body at a deficit to be able to perform physiological processes and support optimal performance. Some studies have shown that nearly 60 percent of female endurance athletes are at risk for LEA and the side effects that come with it (Melin et al. 2015). Sufficient energy availability (EA) or energy balance is defined as having enough dietary energy available to maintain normal physiological functioning after the energy costs of exercise have been met.

To figure out whether you are in an LEA state, you can use the following EA equation.

EA Equation Terms

- *Energy intake (EI):* Total energy (in kilocalories) consumed throughout the day. Relies on self-reporting, tracking, and estimating by the athlete, which can be inaccurate.
- *Exercise energy expenditure (EEE):* Total energy (in kilocalories) burned or expended from exercise throughout the day.
- *Fat-free mass (FFM):* Total body mass, including water, organs, and bones but excluding fat. This is usually measured through body composition testing.

$$EA = EI - EEE / FFM$$

Optimal EA is achieved at 45 kilocalories per kilogram of FFM per day, and less than 30 kilocalories per kilogram of FFM per day is the typical cutoff for optimal physiological function in females. In male athletes, the cutoff for optimal physiological function is unknown.

While there are some downsides to using this equation (such as inaccuracies in food logging and EEE reporting), it can be helpful to examine your habits that could contribute to LEA. Indicators that someone is at a higher risk of LEA include frequently consuming low-calorie, low-sugar foods or stimulants such as caffeine, having a high fiber intake, and eating within a small window of time during the day.

Risk Factors for RED-S

RED-S can occur intentionally or unintentionally depending on the athlete's goals. Intentional RED-S stems from a drive to change body composition or weight, and the restrictive nature of dieting causes a mismatch between energy needs and energy intake. Compulsive RED-S occurs "intentionally" when an individual has a clinically diagnosable eating disorder. Unintentional RED-S happens when an athlete doesn't know they are not matching energy needs to training demands.

While calculations can be done to determine the presence or absence of RED-S, the body is very good at showing symptoms that can lead to a diagnosis of the condition. RED-S can affect every system in the body to a different extent, and knowing some of these signs is important for prevention and recovery. Table 1.8 describes what to look for if you suspect RED-S.

TABLE 1.8   Signs and Symptoms of RED-S

System	Signs and symptoms of RED-S
Endocrine	Low sex hormones; low metabolic hormones such as cortisol, insulin growth factor, leptin, and ghrelin; growth-factor hormones stunting growth
Skeletal	Increased risk of stress fractures due to anabolic effects on bone strength and increases in stress hormones
Hematological	Iron-deficiency anemia
Cardiovascular	Increased cholesterol, heartbeat abnormalities
Immunological	Decreased immune factors leaving the athlete more vulnerable to illness
Gastrointestinal	Dysfunction of the digestive system increasing frequency and severity of diarrhea, constipation, and stomach pains
Psychological	Increased depression and obsessive behaviors

RED-S can have a substantial negative impact on performance, including in the following areas:

- Decreased training adaptations
- Impaired recovery
- Increased injury risk
- Impaired judgment
- Decreased coordination
- Decreased concentration
- Irritability
- Depression
- Decreased glycogen stores
- Decreased muscle strength
- Decreased endurance performance

Adapted from Mountjoy et al. (2023).

RED-S recovery can be relatively straightforward or more complex depending on the root cause. Nutritional habits—particularly overall energy intake, macronutrient consumption, and timing of intake—need to be addressed. Energy deficits must be corrected, and eating more than the predicted energy requirements may be necessary to help jump-start the body's physiological systems. A temporary reduction or complete stoppage of exercise may be necessary depending on the severity of RED-S.

Cognitive behavioral therapy may help an athlete through the recovery process and has been shown to help female athletes regain their menstrual cycles. The use of oral contraceptives to regain the menstrual cycle or improve bone density is not recommended. Transdermal estradiol with cyclic oral progestin can be used temporarily if nutritional, psychological, and lifestyle interventions are not successful. For those with clinical eating disorders, special treatment protocols, including admission to higher levels of care, may be necessary.

Eating Disorders and Disordered Eating

Eating disorders have the highest mortality rate out of all mental health illnesses, and they have a much higher prevalence rate in the sports population, with some studies reporting up to 60 percent of the endurance population suffering from eating disorders and disordered eating (Melin et al. 2015). It is important to note that eating disorders don't discriminate; endurance athletes of any age or gender can develop one.

While everyone faces common risk factors for developing eating disorders—like genetic predisposition, trauma, body dissatisfaction, and a history of controlling nutrition intake—endurance athletes face sport-specific predispositions such as tight-fitting uniforms, pressure from teammates or coaches, and an aesthetic emphasis on leanness. Eating disorders and disordered eating can develop suddenly or over time. Clinical eating disorders are diagnosed using the DSM-5, the standard classification of mental disorders used by mental health professionals in the United States.

Categories of eating disorders include the following:

- *Anorexia nervosa:* Restriction of energy intake well below the needs for exercise and movement, which may or may not lead to low body weight. There is usually body image distortion and an intense fear of gaining weight. Diet is typically very limited due to the fear of carbohydrates and fats.

- *Bulimia nervosa:* Eating a large amount of food in a short period of time and feeling a loss of control, along with other compensatory behaviors (e.g., purging, laxatives, diet pills). An intense fear of gaining weight is also usually present.

- *Binge eating disorder:* Eating large amounts of food without compensatory behaviors once per week for at least three months. Binge episodes are associated with loss of control, rapid eating, and feelings of shame, guilt, and depression.

- *Other specified feeding and eating disorder:* A diagnosis for eating disorders that don't meet the other eating disorder criteria. For example, purging without bingeing or consuming excessive amounts of food after dinner or in the middle of the night.

- *Orthorexia (not formally recognized by the DSM-5):* An obsessive fixation on healthy eating to the point that it damages a person's well-being. For example, eating only clean foods, no sugar, or no processed foods.

Red flags for an eating disorder or disordered eating can vary extensively and can include any or all of the following:

- Decreased concentration, energy, muscle function, coordination, or speed
- Increased fatigue and perceived exertion
- Longer recovery times
- More frequent muscle strains, sprains, fractures, or stress injuries
- Slowed heart rate or blood pressure
- Irregular or missing periods for athletes with ovaries
- Reduced body temperature and increased sensitivity to cold (cold hands and feet)
- Lightheadedness, dizziness, abdominal pain, or gastrointestinal issues such as constipation
- Poorer interaction with coaches or teammates
- Perfectionism
- Increased impatience, crankiness, isolation, introversion, or withdrawal; lack of self-compassion
- Difficulty with days off, rest days, or tapering
- Avoidance of water or liquid calories; excessive water intake
- Preoccupation with own food or other people's food
- Ritualistic eating or avoidance of certain foods
- Excessive concern with body aesthetic
- Extra workouts or exercise beyond what is prescribed
- Concerned reports about an individual by fellow athletes

If you think you or someone you know might have an eating disorder, it is important to get the support you need to recover. A recovery team may consist of a therapist, doctor, and dietitian. If you need support, the National Eating Disorders Association (NEDA), Equip Health, and Within Health are all good resource centers.

Tips for Talking About Eating Disorders

If you are an athlete, a family member of an athlete, or a coach who is trying to figure out how to approach someone you suspect may have an eating disorder, here are some tips for broaching the subject:

- Approach them in a private setting. Call them on the phone or do a video call (e.g., Zoom) if you're not in the same physical location.
- Let them know you are concerned and cite specific reasons why you are concerned about a possible eating disorder.
- Deliver your message directly and precisely and ensure it is relevant, deep, and significant.
- Avoid judging or criticizing. Underfueling can be intentional or unintentional. Disordered eating and eating disorders are mental illnesses that no one chooses to have.
- Make a referral to an appropriate medical provider (therapist, dietitian, doctor, etc.) as soon as possible.
- Know that most people are not going to be excited about seeking help or care. Be prepared for this. They may need to be really encouraged. If you wait until an athlete feels ready, it may be too late (i.e., their health and life could be at risk). Be firm, consistent, and steadfast; otherwise, you may accidentally be colluding with an eating disorder.

Takeaways

- Try not to get caught up in the finer details of nutrition before dialing in your foundational basics like hydrating and eating enough for different days of training.
- Specifying your carbohydrate, protein, and fat types can help you fine-tune your macronutrient intake to optimize performance and recovery.
- Using the athlete's plate model and learning to tune in to hunger and fullness cues can allow you to combine intention with intuition so you aren't left second-guessing if what you are doing is correct.
- RED-S is common in the endurance-athlete population, and it is important to be aware of the signs and symptoms of RED-S so you can prevent it or recover if needed.
- Be aware of the signs and symptoms of eating disorders and disordered eating in case you or someone you know is affected by any of these conditions.

2

SMART USE OF SUPPLEMENTS

I can count on one hand the number of supplements that have helped me as an endurance athlete over the years. The rest were just really expensive urine.

—Amelia Boone, Professional OCR Athlete and Ultra Runner (athlete interview, 2024)

Endurance athletes have been looking to gain an extra edge in competition and training for centuries. Reports of using drugs, foods, and various techniques to gain advantages in sport date back to 776 BC. At that time, Olympians ate certain foods like figs and mushrooms that were believed to benefit their performance (Mathews 2018). More recent reports in the 20th century from sports like cycling involved the use of drugs and performance-enhancing techniques like blood doping to gain that advantage in the Tour de France (Mignon 2003).

In the United States, it wasn't until the Dietary Supplement Health and Education Act of 1994 (DSHEA) that dietary supplements were given a clearer definition: a product "other than tobacco, intended to supplement the diet that contains a vitamin, mineral, herb or botanical, dietary substance, or a concentrate, metabolite, constituent, extract, or combination of the above ingredients; that is intended for ingestion, is not represented as food or as a sole item of a meal or diet, and is labeled as a dietary supplement" (U.S. Congress 1994).

Despite supplements being more well defined, their regulation and roles within sport are less clear. Many countries have some sort of regulatory body that looks at supplements more closely, but these regulations are not always strictly adhered to. In the United States, the Food and Drug Administration (FDA) regulates dietary supplements under a different umbrella than conventional food and drug products. Unfortunately, their purity and guidelines are not very well managed, meaning that the ingredients listed on the label of a supplement may not actually be what is in the supplement. If you choose to take a supplement, know that you are accepting the risk of possible contamination.

To curb unfair use of performance-enhancing substances in the athletic world, the U.S Anti-Doping Agency (USADA) was formed on October 1, 2000, to bring credibility to the anti-doping movement in the United States. It was also implemented as part of the World Anti-Doping Code, which lays out a core set of anti-doping policies that apply throughout the world. To keep athletes up to date, a list of banned substances is published by the World Anti-Doping Agency (WADA) every year for both during and outside of competition season (2024). It is an athlete's responsibility to be aware of banned substances as well as supplement regulations in different countries throughout the world.

According to a 2016 report in the Nutrition Business Journal, it is estimated that sports nutrition supplement sales totaled about $5 billion (2017). Powders, capsules, liquids, and pills are taken specifically to gain an edge. Think about that for a minute. In an industry that is not well regulated, do you want to be the one who gets caught for using a banned substance or has a health interaction with something in a supplement that is not listed on the label? Don't get me wrong; there are

How Can You Use Routine Blood Work as an Endurance Athlete to Determine Deficiencies?

Routine blood work should be an important part of every endurance athlete's annual routine. Think of it like looking under the hood of your car regularly to ensure that something doesn't need fixing. While every endurance athlete should consider their personal history and health conditions when determining what types of blood panels would be good to have drawn, I like to look for the following when working with athletes:

- Full iron panel (serum iron, total iron-binding capacity [TIBC], iron saturation percentage, ferritin)
- Magnesium red blood cell (RBC)
- C-reactive protein (CRP)
- Complete blood count (CBC)
- Vitamin B_{12}
- Vitamin D_3

Outside of this list, things like hormonal labs, full thyroid panels, and electrolytes can be helpful to look at if you have something abnormal going on such as lack of periods, unexplainable fatigue, hair loss, irregular heartbeat, or fainting episodes. It's important in these situations to work with your doctor and dietitian to determine the best panel for you.

some supplements out there that have well-documented research behind them and some companies that go the extra mile with their testing and labeling, but you must be cautious.

When you are considering whether to use a supplement, investigate if the supplement is even necessary for the advantage you are trying to achieve. Do you really need it, or can you achieve the same goal by modifying your diet?

Supplements and sports food products can typically be classified into a few purposeful categories. Evaluating a supplement to see if it fits into one of these categories is a suggested first step in determining whether to supplement:

- Those that contain large amounts of a particular vitamin or mineral to help correct a known deficiency (e.g., vitamin D)
- Those that claim to impact performance directly or indirectly with or without scientific support (e.g., beta-alanine, creatine, caffeine)
- Those that help replenish nutrition in a convenient way (e.g., sports gels or recovery drinks)

Questions When Choosing a New Supplement

Here are some things to ask yourself when choosing a new supplement:

1. Can I get a similar benefit from food?
2. Am I deficient in the nutrients that this supplement provides?
3. Do the risks outweigh the possible benefits?
4. Is the supplement legal and not on the WADA list of prohibited substances?
5. Is this a well-researched supplement? Has it been shown to be effective?
6. Could there be any possible interactions with medications that I take?
7. Is the supplement third-party tested through the National Sanitation Foundation (NSF) program Certified for Sport or through Informed Sport's certification system?

Third-Party Certification

USADA currently only recognizes supplements with the NSF Certified for Sport label. Per its website, NSF is an independent nongovernmental organization whose mission is to improve human health. Certified products get an NSF label after they are tested to confirm they do not contain contaminants, prohibited substances, or masking agents (see figure 2.1).

Per its website, Informed Sport started an international testing and certification program to assure athletes that their supplements were tested for prohibited substances (see figure 2.2).

Remember, even if you see ads from supplement companies or receive advice from well-intentioned family members or coaches who recommend certain products, this does not mean you should consider taking them. You need to make the best choice for yourself to ensure the supplement benefits your unique needs and to avoid potential repercussions.

While it's ideal to try to get nutrition and recovery benefits from food sources, it's not always the most practical. Many endurance athletes feel overwhelmed by the number of supplements out there. Let's talk about which ones might actually be worth your time and money.

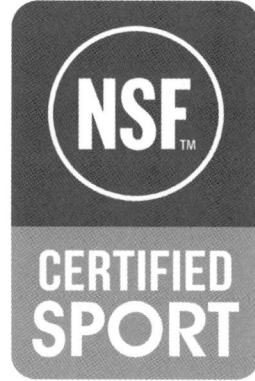

FIGURE 2.1   Certified for Sport label.
Courtesy NSF®.

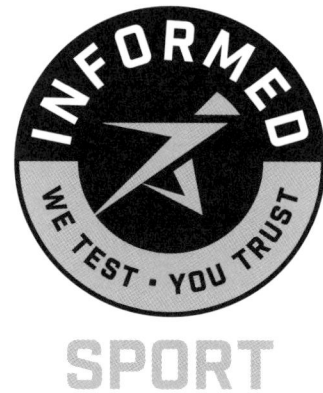

FIGURE 2.2   Informed Sport label.
Courtesy LGC/Informed Sport.

Protein Powders and BCAAs

Are you looking for a quick source of protein to aid recovery and prevent injury? Protein powder can be a very useful way to meet protein goals when struggling to meet nutritional needs due to your schedule or dietary preferences. This could include situations like the following:

- Driving to a training session and needing a quick recovery option postworkout
- Wanting to increase the protein content of baked goods or soups that might otherwise be short
- Wanting to get in protein in the middle of a busy workday when a liquid option might be the best bet
- Being vegetarian or vegan with limited protein options to meet endurance needs

While you could technically use protein powder as your sole source of protein, you could be missing out on key enzymes and nutrients that go along with whole-food sources of protein if you use only protein powder.

Some athletes choose a BCAA supplement for performance reasons. BCAAs include leucine, isoleucine, and valine. They are branched in structure compared to other amino acids and are theorized to induce higher rates of muscle-protein synthesis, act as an alternative source of fuel for the body during endurance exercise, and act as a central nervous system stimulant. In a 2019 meta-analysis, there was no significant effect observed on feelings of central nervous system fatigue with mixed BCAA supplementation; however, it did reduce lactate levels, creatine kinase (CK) levels, glucose, ammonia, and free fatty acids, suggesting that mixed BCAA supplementation during exercise could provide performance benefits (Hormoznejad, Javid, and Mansoori). If you're simply trying to supplement outside of a workout, protein powders already contain varying amounts of mixed BCAAs, so mixed BCAA supplementation on its own may be unnecessary.

Protein powders are concentrated strands of amino acids made from plant and animal products. They can be used creatively to boost the protein content of soups, smoothies, and baked foods or simply mixed in water. While some contain fillers, sweeteners, and flavorings, it is important to try out individual products—some athletes complain about a strong aftertaste.

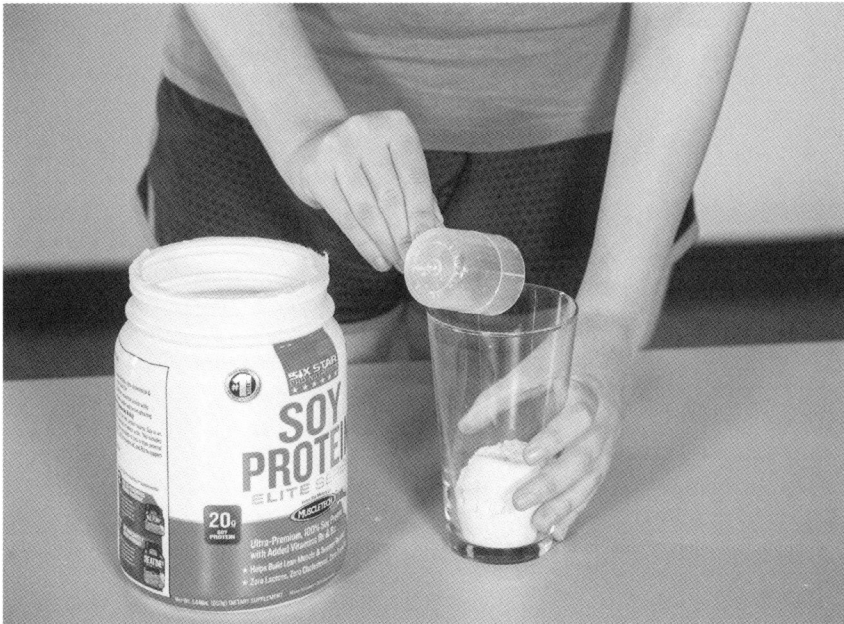

You can add one of the many types of protein powder to your beverages or recipes to help increase your daily protein intake.

Benefits of Protein Powder for Endurance Athletes

Protein powder can be a quick and easy way to increase your overall protein intake in a convenient, low-volume, portable option. Table 2.1 explains how different types of protein powders can be useful for various needs.

TABLE 2.1   Quick Reference Chart for Protein Powders

Protein type	How it is produced	What it is best used for	Possible side effects or downsides
Whey	Watery portion of milk left over after cheese processing. Whey makes up about 20% of milk.	A fast-acting protein source, whey is high in BCAAs, leucine in particular, which can prevent muscle protein breakdown and promote highest recovery rates.	Can cause gas and bloating in sensitive individuals.
Egg	Chicken eggs are dehydrated and ground up.	Easily digested and highest in BCAAs, egg protein is a great choice for recovery and muscle maintenance.	Possible allergen.
Casein	Makes up 80% of milk and is the curd portion that is left over after cheese processing.	Casein digests slower and is effective for maintaining muscle mass and repairing tendon and ligament injuries because it is high in the amino acid proline.	Common allergen.
Rice	Made of ground-up grains of rice. The carbohydrate is separated from the protein in the rice after combining it with an enzyme.	Mildly flavored and more hypoallergenic than other protein powders, rice protein makes a great choice for use in cooking.	Does not contain a complete amino acid profile and is lower in BCAA content.
Pea	Concentrated and extracted from yellow peas.	A great choice for plant-based endurance athletes looking for a protein boost. As a bonus, it contains iron!	Lower amounts of the amino acid methionine. Typically has a stronger taste than other plant protein powders.
Soy	Ground soybeans.	Lower digestibility rate than whey or egg protein powders, but at the top of the plant-based protein powder options for muscle building. Contains a complete amino acid profile.	Possible allergen.
Hemp	Extracted from the hemp plant (not marijuana) and ground up.	Also contains omega-6 and omega-3 fatty acids in addition to its amino acid content.	Higher fiber content, which can lead to gas and bloating.
Collagen	Ground-up animal bone, skin, and cartilage.	Three types (I, II, and III) are found in supplemental protein powder. Supports organs and soft tissues. Can be particularly useful for tendon and ligament support.	Not an option for vegans or vegetarians.

Iron

Iron is a crucial mineral for endurance athletes because of its key role in producing energy and transporting oxygen throughout the body. More specifically, not getting enough iron may hinder aerobic power and the body's ability to obtain physiological adaptations to exercise training. A 2019 review by Sim et al. illustrated that iron deficiency affects about 15 to 35 percent of female athletes and 5 to 11 percent of male athletes and identified the main causes of iron deficiency as being related to gastro-intestinal losses, menstrual cycles, exercise hemolysis (foot striking the ground), nonsteroidal anti-inflammatory drug (NSAID) use, sweating, and LEA.

Iron-deficiency anemia is one of many types of anemia. The definition of anemia is not having enough of certain nutrients to produce healthy red blood cells. With iron-deficiency anemia, if the body does not have enough iron available, it will pull from its iron stores, otherwise known as ferritin. Common symptoms of iron-deficiency anemia include fatigue, poor exercise performance, difficulty concentrating, inadequate temperature regulation (cold), lightheadedness, and brittle nails. See table 2.2 for explanations of the three stages of iron-deficiency anemia.

TABLE 2.2 The Three Stages of Iron-Deficiency Anemia

Stage I (iron deficiency)	Ferritin <35 µg/L
	Hb >115 g/L
	Transferrin saturation >16%
	Performance may not be impacted yet, but iron levels may need to be corrected.
Stage II (iron-deficiency nonanemia)	Ferritin <20 µg/L
	Hb >115 g/L
	Transferrin saturation <16%
	Some performance impact.
Stage III (iron-deficiency anemia)	Ferritin < 12 µg/L
	Hb <115 g/L
	Transferrin saturation<16%
	Severe performance impact.

Adapted based on guidelines by Sim et al. (2019).

Benefits of Iron Supplementation for Endurance Athletes

Iron supplementation with pills or, in severe cases, iron infusions may be required for endurance athletes to get out of an iron-deficiency anemia state. Supplements allow athletes to take in a consistent and high amount of iron that they may otherwise not be able to get from their diet. While supplementation can be helpful, it is important for endurance athletes to evaluate the causes(s) of their low iron availability to determine a holistic approach to long-term iron level maintenance.

Troubleshooting Chronic Low Ferritin: A Holistic Athlete Approach

If an endurance athlete struggles with chronic low ferritin, there are several areas to explore to determine if there is a greater issue that needs to be addressed. Consider the following:

- *Gastrointestinal bleeding:* This problem needs to be addressed by a gastrointestinal specialist and will require a colonoscopy to get an inside look at what is going on.

- *Underfueling:* Not consuming enough iron from food on a regular basis will require an athlete to get enough iron to maintain stasis from outside sources (see recommendation in table 2.3 for daily iron requirements from food sources).

- *Micronutrient consumption:* The pathway that stores iron and produces energy relies on a number of micronutrients to run smoothly. The specific micronutrients required for iron transport, utilization, and storage are vitamin A (retinol), copper (bioavailable), magnesium, and vitamin C. Without these micronutrients, this process can be interrupted or stopped overall, and iron can essentially get stuck in intestinal cells.
  - Examples of copper-rich foods (recommended intake is 1 mcg/day): potatoes, dark chocolate, mushrooms, chickpeas, and oysters
  - Examples of foods rich in vitamin A (retinol): butter, beef liver, and cod liver oil
  - Examples of foods rich in vitamin C: strawberries, bell peppers, potatoes, and cruciferous vegetables
  - Examples of magnesium-rich foods: nuts, seeds, leafy greens, and dark chocolate

- *Possible pathogens:* While this may not be your first consideration, it is important to consider the impact of digestive pathogens such as fungal overgrowth (candida), small intestine bacterial overgrowth (SIBO), and *H. pylori*, which can sequester iron from the system and use it for their own fuel.

- *Heavy periods:* Unusually heavy periods every month can cause significant blood loss. If this is something you struggle with, make sure to address it with your ob-gyn to understand the underlying hormonal causes of such large amounts of blood loss.

Considerations for Iron Supplementation

You should have blood work done, including measuring your ferritin, hemoglobin, and iron transferrin saturation levels, before engaging in iron supplementation. You should also evaluate your dietary iron intake before supplementing iron. The recommended reference daily intake (RDI) of elemental iron for the general population is 8 mg per day for males and 18 mg per day for females. Due to increased losses for endurance athletes related to foot strike hemolysis and sweat, it is likely that intake should be higher for the endurance population; however, no standard has been established.

The timing and form of iron being consumed are important factors to consider when evaluating overall dietary iron intake. As demonstrated in a 2000 study by Beard and Tobin, heme sources of iron (from meat) are absorbed at a rate of 5 to 35 percent on average, while nonheme sources of iron (from plants) are absorbed at a rate of 2 to 20 percent on average during a meal. Consuming vitamin C at the same time as both heme and nonheme iron sources can increase iron absorption, while eating foods containing calcium, phytates, and polyphenol along with iron can inhibit nonheme iron absorption.

If you are looking to obtain iron from food sources, the list of foods containing high amounts of iron in table 2.3 may be helpful.

TABLE 2.3   **High-Iron Foods**

Food source	Amount of iron per serving
Canned clams (3 oz [90 g])	23.8 mg
Fortified cereal (1/2 cup)	9-12 mg
Soybeans (1/2 cup [115 g])	4 mg
Pumpkin seeds (1 oz [30 g])	4 mg
White beans (1/2 cup [115 g])	4 mg
Spinach (1 cup [30 g] raw)	3 mg
Pork (3 oz [90 g])	2.7 mg
Soy milk (1 cup [240 mL])	2.7 mg
Ground beef (3 oz [90 g])	2.2 mg
Cashews (1 oz [35 g])	1.6 mg

Data from Academy of Nutrition and Dietetics (2018).

How to Supplement

When considering iron supplementation, think about the timing of the supplement you are taking. The liver produces a hormone called hepcidin, which regulates the body's ability to recycle or absorb iron and can block iron absorption altogether. According to a study by McCormick et al. in 2020, hepcidin levels rise throughout the day and with inflammation levels, reaching a peak three to six hours after training. Therefore, the best time to take an iron supplement may be in the morning or 30 minutes after a morning workout.

For athletes with a sensitive stomach, research indicates that supplementing every other day may be just as effective as supplementing every day and can help reduce gastrointestinal stress. Oral supplementation of iron comes in liquid or tablet form. Ferrous forms of iron supplementation (fumarate, sulfate, and gluconate) are the most common; however, these may cause gastrointestinal distress (Brittenham 2018).

As demonstrated by Dawson et al. in 2006, iron supplement amounts of around 100 milligrams per day tend to have a positive effect on ferritin levels when administered for 8 to 12 weeks. However, this depends on gastrointestinal tolerance and may require an every-other-day supplementation strategy.

This apple cinnamon smoothie recipe is high in iron.

Apple Cinnamon Smoothie

This recipe provides 7 mg of iron per serving, making it a great choice for athletes who are low in iron.
Servings: 1

Ingredients
- 1-1/4 cup (300 mL) oat milk
- 1 small apple, cored and chopped
- 1/2 cup (100 g) cauliflower rice (or chopped florets)
- 1/4 cup (30 g) vanilla protein powder
- 1/4 tsp cinnamon
- 1 tbsp chia seeds (plus more for garnish if desired)

Directions
Place all ingredients in blender and blend.

Vitamin D

Vitamin D is a fat-soluble vitamin that can be obtained from limited food sources (see table 2.4), supplementation, and sun exposure. It plays key interactive roles with over 1,000 genes in the body. For endurance athletes, vitamin D is significant not only for bone strength but also for immune health, inflammation, and skeletal growth and recovery. Maintaining adequate vitamin D levels is an important way to avoid injury and illness and to optimize athlete performance.

Benefits of Vitamin D for Endurance Athletes

Maintaining optimal vitamin D levels is essential for endurance athletes to stay healthy and injury-free. Some of vitamin D's more well-known functions include bone health promotion, immune system regulation, insulin management, and blood pressure regulation.

- *Bone health:* Along with calcium, magnesium, and vitamin K, vitamin D plays a key role in bone resorption. More specifically, it helps absorb calcium to maintain bone mineral density. Bone health can be directly related to stress-fracture risk, which is key to staying healthy in endurance-athlete populations. In a 2012 study by Sonneville et al. on adolescent girls in the United States, those with the highest levels of vitamin D intake were at the lowest risk of stress fracture, while another study conducted in 2016 by Miller et al. found that 83 percent of those experiencing a stress fracture had vitamin D levels below 40 nanograms per milliliter.

- *Immune support:* Vitamin D plays an important role in the immune system's ability to regulate inflammation and respond properly to acute illnesses. Keeping vitamin D levels sufficient can help fight off infectious diseases before they start (Wacker and Holick 2013).

- *Insulin function:* Vitamin D has demonstrated inflammation-balancing properties, which could reduce the risk of insulin resistance. It also stimulates the release of insulin directly; as a result, low levels can impact blood glucose control (Sung et al. 2012).

- *Blood pressure:* While the physiological processes of vitamin D and blood pressure are still not fully understood, it is hypothesized that low vitamin D can contribute to higher levels of vascular stiffness and affect calcium and parathyroid production, resulting in higher blood pressure levels (Jensen et al. 2023).

The gold standard for determining vitamin D status is to look at circulating amounts of calcidiol (25-hydroxyvitamin D_3 [$25(OH)D_3$]) concentration. There is debate in the medical community as to what levels of vitamin D are optimal. According to the U.S. Endocrine Society as outlined in a 2011 study by Holick et al., vitamin D insufficiency is determined to be less than 30 nanograms per milliliter. However, some sports medicine professionals recommend an optimal level for athletes of 50 nanograms per milliliter.

Considerations for Vitamin D Supplementation and How to Supplement

Vitamin D stands out on the spectrum of vitamins because it cannot be obtained from many food sources. More traditionally, vitamin D is considered a hormone that is made active by sun exposure to UVB rays. Endurance athletes often wrongly assume that because they exercise outside, they will be able to produce all their vitamin D from the sun. This simply isn't the case; many factors influence the body's ability to produce sufficient amounts of vitamin D, including the season, the latitude, your sunscreen use, your clothing choices, and the amount of melanin in your skin.

Holick et al. recommend supplementing with 1,500 to 2,000 international units (IU) of vitamin D_3 per day when sufficient exposure to sunlight is not available (2011). Higher doses may be required if an athlete has a deficiency, is taking a medication that affects vitamin D absorption (such as antacids, laxatives, or cholesterol-lowering medications), or possesses a genetic variant that may affect absorption. In this case, under medical supervision, the athlete could undergo a high-dose loading protocol of 10,000 IU of vitamin D_3 per day for 8 to 10 weeks.

More is not necessarily better when supplementing vitamin D because it is fat soluble and able to be stored in body tissues. This is why it is very important to look at your current vitamin D levels and be supervised by a professional when considering supplementation. At-home UV light therapy lamps may be a useful alternative to help raise vitamin D levels, but research is unclear on how beneficial they can be. Refer to table 2.4 for common foods containing vitamin D.

TABLE 2.4   Foods that Contain High Amounts of Vitamin D

Food source	Amount of vitamin D per serving
Fatty fish (salmon)	383-570 IU (3 oz [90 g])
Egg yolk	37 IU (1 large yolk)
Fortified milk and soy milk	80 IU (1 cup [240 mL])
Irradiated mushrooms	114-1,140 IU (1 cup [80-100 g])
Yogurt	116 IU (1 cup [230 g])
Fortified fruit juices	100 IU (1 cup [240 mL])

Data from U.S. Department of Agriculture (2015).

Magnesium

A catalyst for over 300 processes in the body, magnesium plays a key role in muscle contraction, energy metabolism, protein synthesis, and blood pressure regulation. A magnesium deficiency can have a profound effect on an endurance athlete's inflammation levels and muscular recovery rates due to higher levels of oxidative stress. It can also influence the body's ability to make enough ATP to power training sessions. And for endurance athletes with a history of bone issues, it plays a key role in bone strength and long-term bone health.

Magnesium can be found naturally in a number of different food sources; however, research indicates that more than 60 percent of the population fails to consume the recommended dietary allowance (RDA) of magnesium (Reno et al. 2022). Refer to table 2.5 for a list of common foods containing magnesium.

TABLE 2.5   Magnesium-Rich Foods

Food source	Amount of magnesium per serving
Pumpkin seed kernels (1 oz [30 g])	168 mg
Almonds (1 oz [30 g])	80 mg
Spinach (1/2 cup [22 g], boiled)	78 mg
Cashews (1 oz [35 g])	74 mg
Peanuts (1/4 cup [30 g])	63 mg
Soy milk (1 cup [240 mL])	61 mg
Black beans (1/2 cup [115 g], cooked)	60 mg
Edamame (1/2 cup [115 g], shelled)	50 mg
Dark chocolate (1 oz [30 g], 60-69% cacao)	50 mg
Smooth peanut butter (2 tbsp)	49 mg
Whole wheat bread (2 slices)	46 mg
Avocado (1 cup [230 g])	44 mg
Baked potato (3.5 oz [105 g])	43 mg
Brown rice (1/2 cup [115 g], cooked)	42 mg
Plain yogurt (1/2 cup [115 g])	42 mg
Banana (1 medium)	32 mg
Atlantic salmon (3 oz [90 g], farmed)	26 mg
Raisins (1/2 cup [80 g])	23 mg

Data from "Magnesium Consumer Factsheet," National Institute of Mental Health, last updated March 22, 2021, https://ods.od.nih.gov/factsheets/Magnesium-Consumer/.

Benefits of Magnesium for Endurance Athletes

Endurance athletes have higher magnesium needs than the average person because of increased energy needs during exercise, increased sweat loss, and increased physiological stress. The benefits of magnesium for endurance athletes are many and affect energy, performance, and muscle recovery.

• *Reduced muscle soreness:* In a 2022 study published by Reno et al., recreational strength-based athletes had a significant decrease in muscle soreness and rate of perceived effort (RPE) when they were supplementing with 350 milligrams of magnesium daily. This result has been replicated in other studies that have shown reduced markers of CK, an indicator of muscle damage (Córdova et al. 2019). By attenuating delayed-onset muscle soreness with proper magnesium intake, endurance athletes may be able to recover more quickly and train harder and at higher volumes.

• *Sleep benefits:* Magnesium deficiency can affect overall circadian rhythm and melatonin production. Studies on magnesium's effect on sleep quality are limited; however, Abbasi et al. demonstrated in a 2012 trial that magnesium supplementation in the elderly decreased cortisol levels, increased melatonin concentration, and decreased insomnia. These findings suggest a possible solution for athletes who struggle with sleep and want to use more natural sleep aids to improve sleep quantity and quality.

How to Supplement

According to the National Institutes of Health (NIH), the recommended daily magnesium intake is 400 to 420 milligrams for adult males and 300 to 360 milligrams for adult females (2021). However, endurance athletes may need more because they lose the mineral in urine and sweat. As a reminder, even a small deficiency can negatively affect exercise performance and oxidative stress levels. If an athlete does not truly have a magnesium deficiency, though, supplementation may not be necessary (Nielsen and Lukaski 2006). There is no standard recommendation for magnesium supplementation, although some studies have indicated that using 350 to 500 milligrams per day produces benefits for those who are deficient. Table 2.6 compares specific types of magnesium supplements and their main uses.

TABLE 2.6   Comparing Types of Magnesium Supplements and Their Uses

Form of magnesium	Main use
Magnesium citrate	Laxative
Magnesium oxide	Laxative
Magnesium threonate	Higher absorption rate, brain health, sleep
Magnesium hydroxide (also known as milk of magnesia)	Laxative
Magnesium glycinate	Higher absorption rate, muscle health, sleep

Adapted from K. Berkheiser, "How Much Magnesium Should You Take Per Day?" Healthline, last modified November 13, 2023, https://www.healthline.com/nutrition/magnesium-dosage.

The following magnesium-rich smoothie bowl recipe can be a great addition to an endurance athlete's diet if they need more magnesium.

Vanilla Berry Pumpkin Seed Smoothie Bowl

Each smoothie bowl contains about 400 mg of magnesium, making it a great choice to boost your intake of this mineral that is lost in high amounts through sweat.

Ingredients

- 1-1/2 cup (360 mL) soy milk
- 1 scoop vanilla protein powder
- 1/2 cup (72.5 g) frozen blueberries
- 1/2 cup (75 g) frozen strawberries
- 1 tbsp almond butter
- 1 tbsp pumpkin seeds (for topping)
- 1 tbsp coconut flakes (for topping)
- 2 tbsp chia seeds (for topping)

Directions

1. Add all ingredients except pumpkin seeds, chia seeds, and coconut flakes to a blender. Blend until smooth.
2. Pour smoothie into a bowl and sprinkle on toppings (chia seeds, pumpkin seeds, and coconut flakes). Enjoy!

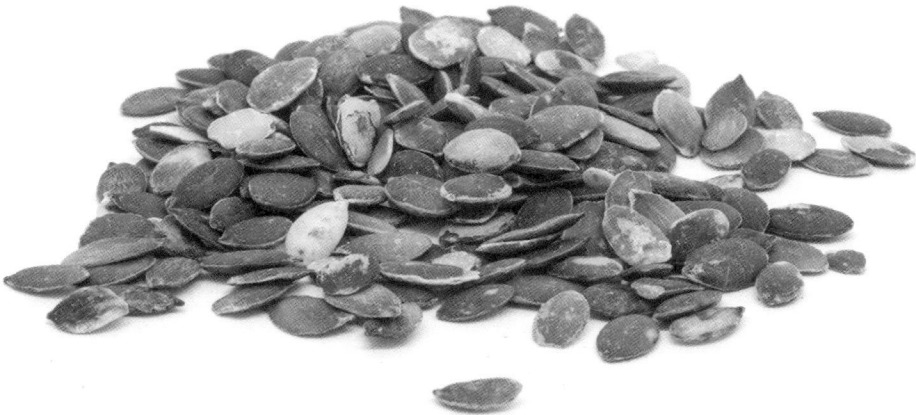

Melanie Hobson / EyeEm/Getty Images

Pumpkin seeds are a key source of magnesium.

Beta-Alanine

Beta-alanine is a nonessential amino acid whose highest amounts are found in meat, poultry, and fish. It works together with the amino acid histidine to increase overall levels of the dipeptide carnosine in the body. Carnosine is stored in the brain and muscles, and it plays an antioxidant role and buffers acidity (hydrogen ions, or H^+ ions) during higher intensity exercise sessions. This is how carnosine works during exercise:

1. Glucose is broken down and used for energy production, creating lactic acid as a by-product.
2. Lactic acid is converted into lactate, which produces more H^+ ions and creates an acidic environment in the muscles.
3. This acidic environment causes the muscles to become more fatigued.
4. Carnosine comes in and buffers these H^+ ions, allowing for increased exercise capacity.

Possible Benefits of Beta-Alanine for Endurance Athletes

Beta-alanine presents itself as an amino acid capable of helping endurance athletes reduce fatigue and increase their ability to train harder. At this time, beta-alanine has mostly been studied for increased anaerobic benefits, not aerobic endurance benefits.

- *Fatigue reduction:* During exercise, particularly anaerobic exercise, H^+ ions are produced in muscles, increasing the acidity. These H^+ ions can decrease the body's ability to use glucose, which can, in turn, increase muscular fatigue. Carnosine production in the muscle (increased by supplementing beta-alanine) can buffer H^+ ions and prevent muscular fatigue during high-intensity exercise like short intervals of one to four minutes or high bursts of intensity in longer endurance events (Hobson et al. 2012).

- *Potential to increase training capacity:* Beta-alanine may increase endurance athletes' ability to train hard by reducing the damage caused by high levels of muscle acidity.

How to Supplement

Beta-alanine is best used in a loading fashion with a recommended dose of two to six grams per day for two to four weeks. Once the initial loading phase is complete, the dosage can be cut in half to maintain muscle carnosine levels. You don't need to take it at any particular time of the day, but excessive supplementation (more than 800 milligrams) at one time can cause a tingling sensation (i.e., paresthesia) in the face and hands. To avoid this, you can split up the dose throughout the day or use the patented slow-release form, CarnoSyn (Harris, Jones, and Wise 2008). Current recommendations suggest that beta-alanine supplementation is safe for athlete use.

Omega-3 Fatty Acids

Omega-3 polyunsaturated fatty acids (n-3 PUFAs) are considered essential because of the body's inability to produce enough of them to support regular functioning. There are three types of n-3 PUFAs: eicosapentaenoic acid (EPA), docosahexaenoic acid (DHA), and α-linolenic acid (ALA*). EPA and DHA are the n-3 PUFAs that are mainly responsible for health benefits. Their main function in the body is making up the cellular membranes of the brain, heart, immune system, and skeletal muscle.

The majority of dietary EPA and DHA comes from fish products, but small amounts can be found in eggs and organic meats. Common plant-based ALA sources include walnuts, flax, and chia seeds.

Benefits of Omega-3 Fatty Acids for Endurance Athletes

Omega-3 fatty acids have been shown to have positive impacts on health and performance, specifically for endurance athletes, including balancing inflammation, enhancing muscle recovery, and bolstering immune support.

- *Inflammation balance and enhanced exercise recovery:* The most common reason for endurance athletes to supplement omega-3s is for their inflammation-balancing properties. However, it is important to keep in mind that not all inflammation is bad. In fact, some inflammation after exercise may be necessary for important training adaptations to occur and the body to repair and regenerate (Cerqueira et al. 2020). Consider the training session's intensity and duration when deciding whether to use an inflammation-balancing supplement like omega-3s after exercise. When appropriate, omega-3s have been shown to reduce muscle soreness and oxidative stress, which allows an endurance athlete to recover faster (Heaton et al. 2017).

---

*ALA can be converted to EPA and DHA; however, the conversion rate is relatively low at an average of 3 percent in males and 10 percent in females (Philpott, Witard, and Galloway 2019).

- *Immune support:* Several studies have demonstrated that omega-3 supplementation after exercise can upregulate key immune-modulating factors such as interleukins and natural killer cells and lead to fewer incidences of upper respiratory tract infections (Heaton et al. 2017). More research needs to be done in this area, but these preliminary studies offer evidence that omega-3 supplementation may be beneficial to endurance athletes engaging in stressful training blocks that could suppress the immune system.

How to Supplement

Unfortunately, there is currently no clear consensus on an omega-3 supplementation recommendation for endurance athletes. However, in a study of elite Olympic athletes conducted by Drobnic et al. in 2017, a dose-dependent increase in omega-3 levels was seen with the use of 1.5 to 3 grams per day for a 16-week period.

There are several different forms of omega-3 supplements out there, so choosing the most bioavailable form may be beneficial. The four types of omega-3 supplements are ethyl ester, phospholipid, triglyceride, and free fatty acid. Based on available information from research done by Schuchardt and Hahn (2013), the triglyceride form is the most bioavailable and cost-effective type on the market (2013).

Refer to table 2.7 for foods rich in omega-3 fatty acids.

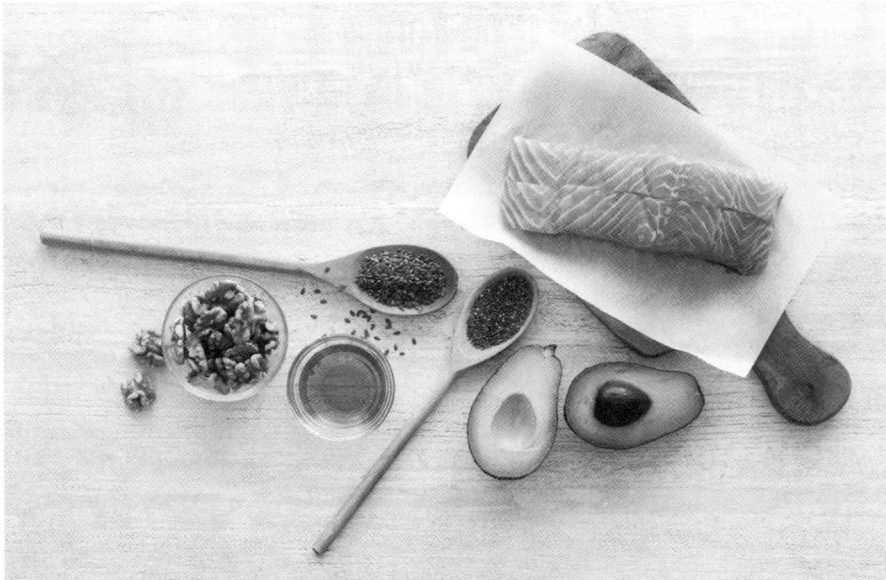

SCIENCE PHOTO LIBRARY/Science Photo Library RF/Getty Images

Foods rich in Omega-3 fatty acids include salmon, avocado, walnuts, chia seeds, flax seeds, and canola oil.

TABLE 2.7 Foods Rich in Omega-3 Fatty Acids

Omega-3 foods and portion sizes	Amount of total EPA or DHA per serving
Salmon (3 oz [90 g])	1.7 g
Trout (3 oz [90 g])	0.8 g
Oysters (3 oz [90 g])	0.5 g
Canned tuna (3 oz [90 g])	0.3 g
Shrimp (3 oz [90 g])	0.2 g
Spirulina (1 tbsp)	0.2 g
Seaweed (1 oz [30 g])	0.2 g
Omega-3 milk (8 oz [240 mL])	0.05 g

USDA Foods Database.

Omega-3 Supplement Labels

The labels on omega-3 supplements can be misleading, so it is important to be able to decipher them and choose a supplement with appropriate amounts of EPA or DHA (see figure 2.3).

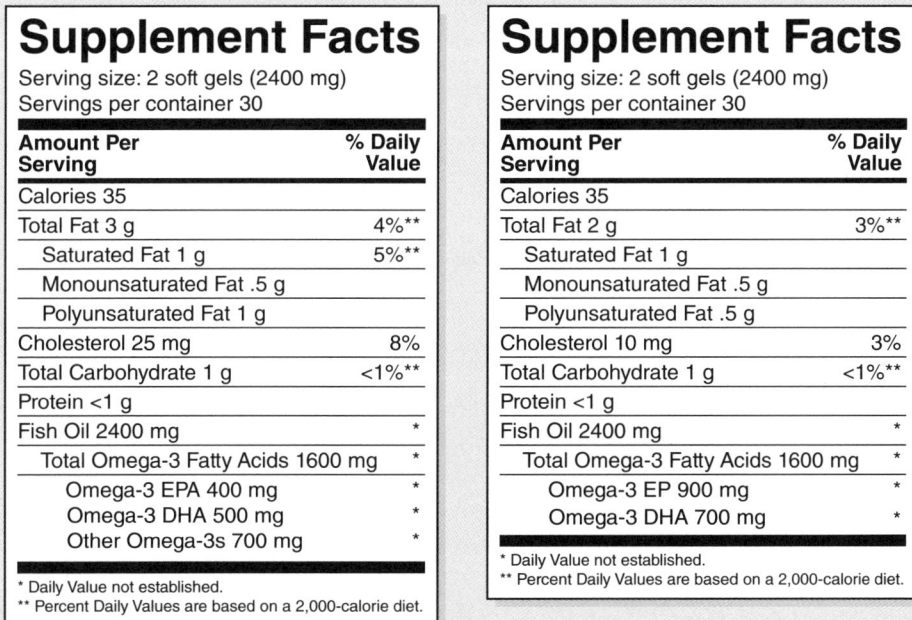

Supplement Facts

Serving size: 2 soft gels (2400 mg)
Servings per container 30

Amount Per Serving	% Daily Value
Calories 35	
Total Fat 3 g	4%**
Saturated Fat 1 g	5%**
Monounsaturated Fat .5 g	
Polyunsaturated Fat 1 g	
Cholesterol 25 mg	8%
Total Carbohydrate 1 g	<1%**
Protein <1 g	
Fish Oil 2400 mg	*
Total Omega-3 Fatty Acids 1600 mg	*
Omega-3 EPA 400 mg	*
Omega-3 DHA 500 mg	*
Other Omega-3s 700 mg	*

* Daily Value not established.
** Percent Daily Values are based on a 2,000-calorie diet.

Supplement Facts

Serving size: 2 soft gels (2400 mg)
Servings per container 30

Amount Per Serving	% Daily Value
Calories 35	
Total Fat 2 g	3%**
Saturated Fat 1 g	
Monounsaturated Fat .5 g	
Polyunsaturated Fat .5 g	
Cholesterol 10 mg	3%
Total Carbohydrate 1 g	<1%**
Protein <1 g	
Fish Oil 2400 mg	*
Total Omega-3 Fatty Acids 1600 mg	*
Omega-3 EP 900 mg	*
Omega-3 DHA 700 mg	*

* Daily Value not established.
** Percent Daily Values are based on a 2,000-calorie diet.

FIGURE 2.3 Two different Omega-3 fish oil supplements and examples of how the label may be deceiving when looking at total EPA and DHA content.

Creatine

Creatine and endurance athletes are not typically thought of together. In fact, creatine is often associated with power sports and muscle building. While it's true that creatine can promote better output and strength in power-related sports, endurance athletes may be able to benefit from its use as well.

Creatine is a nonprotein amino acid compound found mainly in meat products and seafood. After it is consumed, the body stores it intramuscularly as phosphocreatine or as free creatine. About half your required creatine comes from food and supplementation, while the other half is made in the liver and kidneys from arginine, methionine, and glycine. See table 2.8 for a list of creatine-rich foods.

TABLE 2.8   **Creatine-Rich Foods**

Food source	Average amount of creatine per oz
Beef	0.14 g
Pork	0.13 g
Salmon	0.12 g
Chicken	0.12 g
Turkey	0.10 g

Adapted from Bakian et al. (2020).

Benefits of Creatine for Endurance Athletes

Creatine plays many roles in the body, though its most well-known purpose is to maintain energy availability during power sports and quick-burst exercises. It does this in something called the *phosphagen creatine system*, where creatine works in combination with a phosphoryl group to resynthesize ATP, producing energy to keep muscles performing.

- *Enhanced recovery:* In a 2004 study performed by Santos et al., marathon runners were given a creatine-loading protocol before a 30K race. After the race, their inflammation-marker levels were significantly decreased, which decreased excessive oxidative stress—something that could lead to increased injury risk—and potentially allowed endurance athletes to recover and resume normal training activities quicker.

- *Increased heat tolerance:* While not all endurance athletes live in hot climates, having a tool to tolerate heat while training or racing could prevent waning performance. Several studies have demonstrated that creatine supplementation produces a better thermoregulatory response (e.g., heart rate, sweat rate) during prolonged exercise in the heat (Kreider et al. 2017).

• *Increased glycogen storage rates:* Glycogen, or carbohydrate stored in the muscle and liver, is a key powerhouse for endurance exercise. Your body typically has about 90 minutes' to 2 hours' worth of carbohydrate stored to power endurance exercise before it turns to other sources such as fat, protein, and outside sources of carbohydrate for energy production. While creatine supplementation by itself does not increase glycogen storage rates, when creatine is combined with carbohydrate intake, glycogen storage rates increase compared to carbohydrate intake alone (Nelson et al. 2001). Increased glycogen storage rates could allow an endurance athlete to power through back-to-back training sessions better without as much of a performance impact.

• *Increased exercise capacity:* Several studies have demonstrated that creatine loading can increase time to exhaustion during supramaximal workloads. This mechanism can be attributed to creatine's ability to delay anaerobic glycolysis and decrease the accumulation of H^+ ions and ammonia in the muscles and blood (Stout et al. 2000).

How to Supplement

The body degrades 1 to 2 percent of its stored creatine each day, which means that you must restore about 1 to 3 grams of creatine daily to maintain sufficient levels (60 to 80 percent full intramuscularly). About half of this should be consumed through food or supplementation, and the other half will be supplied by the liver and kidneys. For reference, 1 pound (0.5 kilograms) of meat contains an average of 1 to 2 grams of creatine (see table 2.8). Therefore, to top off intramuscular creatine stores, supplementation can help make up that difference. Because vegetarian and vegan athletes don't consume animal products, they may benefit more from creatine supplementation.

If you are considering creatine supplementation, here are a few things to note:

1. *The form of the supplement:* There are many forms of supplemental creatine, but the most researched and bioavailable is creatine monohydrate. Peak absorption of creatine monohydrate occurs about 60 minutes after taking the supplement and drops after that.

2. *Dosage and loading:* Creatine loading is not necessary to gain benefits. Daily supplementation of 3 to 5 grams will produce benefits, but it will take longer to see the effects. If you desire quicker results, an initial loading period of 3 grams per kilogram of body weight for five to seven days can fill up your creatine stores. After that, supplementing with 3 to 5 grams of creatine per day can maintain those store levels.

3. *Carbohydrate intake:* Consuming high amounts of carbohydrate along with a creatine supplement may improve absorption and storage

of both creatine and glycogen in the muscle. Therefore, it may be beneficial to take your creatine supplement with a carbohydrate source like fruit, whole grains, or sweetened nut milk.

4. *Health concerns from supplementation:* Unsubstantiated claims have been made about creatine supplementation causing renal dysfunction, muscle cramping, and gastrointestinal distress. None of these claims have been backed up by studies; in fact, many of these conditions have actually been improved with the use of creatine supplementation (Krieder et al. 2017).

Caffeine

Caffeine is one of the most commonly used "drugs" or supplements in the world and has been shown to increase mental alertness, improve mood, and enhance exercise performance. Caffeine can be ingested in many forms, including gum, coffee, tea, tablets, and even sports nutrition products such as gels and hydration mixes (see table 2.9).

Caffeine metabolism is individualized, and genetic variations (specifically the CYP1A2 and ADORA2A genes) can affect how each athlete absorbs, metabolizes, and uses caffeine. Consume caffeine cautiously because it can increase issues such as anxiety and sleep inhibition (Guest et al. 2021).

TABLE 2.9   Caffeine Content of Common Food and Sports Nutrition Products

Food or sports nutrition product and portion	Amount of caffeine per serving
Coca-Cola (8 oz [240 mL])	22 mg
Green tea (8 oz [240 mL])	28 mg
Black tea (8 oz [240 mL])	47 mg
Run Gum caffeinated gum (1 piece)	50 mg
Shot of espresso (1 oz [30 mL])	64 mg
Red Bull energy drink (8 oz [240 mL])	68 mg
Maurten caffeinated gel (1 gel)	100 mg

Benefits of Caffeine for Endurance Athletes

One of the most studied performance enhancers on the market, caffeine is one of the few supplements that has been actually shown to make a significant difference for reducing fatigue and perceived effort for endurance athletes. Use of caffeine must be personalized, but its benefits could help endurance athletes make an untapped jump in race performance.

- *Reduced fatigue:* Caffeine reduces fatigue because of the effects it has on the central nervous system (CNS) by blocking adenosine from binding to its receptors (Guest et al. 2021). Normally, adenosine acts as a brake for the brain, inducing sleepiness and fatigue.

- *Reduced perceived effort:* Caffeine has led to observed improvements in both pain perception and RPE. A meta-analysis of 21 studies demonstrated a 5.6 percent reduction in RPE and 11 percent improvement in performance with caffeine supplementation (Doherty and Smith 2005). Caffeine appears to do this by increasing hormonelike substances in the brain called beta-endorphins, which reduce pain perception.

- *Increased cognition when sleep-deprived:* In studies done on special forces, caffeine consumption maintained or enhanced cognitive function on little to no sleep (Guest et al. 2021). This benefit could allow endurance athletes who are racing at night or over long distances to continue without as many side effects of sleep deprivation.

How to Supplement

According to a 2018 meta-analysis by Southward, Rutherfurd-Markwick, and Ali, caffeine taken in moderate doses before exercise can help improve performance. A dose of 3 to 6 milligrams per kilogram of body weight is recommended, but 6 milligrams per kilogram of body weight may not offer additional benefits over 3 milligrams per kilogram of body weight. Dosage depends on the athlete's responses to caffeine and should be trialed in varying amounts to see what works best. Keep in mind that more is not necessarily better when it comes to caffeine ingestion; it can actually impair performance if taken at too high amounts. Peak concentrations of caffeine reach the blood within one hour of ingestion, which is important to know for timing your supplementation before and during exercise sessions.

Because of its ability to reduce fatigue and increase carbohydrate oxidation, similar doses of caffeine may be used during exercise. However, caffeine also increases gastrointestinal stimulation and can cause jitteriness, so use caution. It may be beneficial for an endurance athlete to use a product such as caffeinated gum to reduce the risk of gastrointestinal distress. Caffeinated gum allows caffeine to absorb into the bloodstream quicker and does not appear to directly cause gastrointestinal stimulation.

What About a Caffeine Taper Before a Target Event?

A 2019 study by Lara et al. demonstrated that consistent caffeine consumption created some progressive tolerance but that performance benefits were still present over a 20-day period, suggesting that abstaining from caffeine before an event could produce a more significant performance enhancement before a big effort. Unfortunately, habitual caffeine consumers who abstain may experience jitters, headaches, anxiety, and fatigue, which could offer more negatives than positives before a target event.

Beet Juice

You may have heard that beets are the hottest new supplement for endurance athletes, but what makes this root vegetable superior to all others? Beets are rich in dietary nitrates, but not the kind you might think of as food preservatives. Nitrates themselves don't do much in the body, but after ingestion, dietary nitrates from beets are converted into nitric oxide; the process begins in the mouth and progresses to the stomach. Nitric oxide is considered a vasodilator, meaning it allows blood vessels to relax and more oxygen to be transported to the working muscles (i.e., it lowers the oxygen demand during exercise). In turn, this helps the mitochondria generate energy and improves the efficiency of muscle contraction.

Benefits of Beet Juice for Endurance Athletes

Consuming beet juice may help endurance athletes increase oxygen capacity, improve muscle contraction, reduce inflammation, and produce energy. What does this mean for you? Ultimately, it means you could have less muscle fatigue, less energy required to perform endurance exercise, more oxygen delivered to your muscles, and improved recovery time.

How to Supplement

Studies have shown that 300 to 1,041 milligrams of dietary nitrate supplementation is needed to produce performance-enhancing effects (Macuh and Knap 2021). Intake appears to be most effective two to three hours before the intended start of exercise. It is important to note that differences have been observed in the amount of beet juice needed for performance enhancement for well-trained versus everyday endurance athletes. Rokkedal-Lausch et al. published a study in 2019 demonstrating that elite athletes may need a higher and more prolonged dosage of beet juice to experience the same effects as the everyday athlete and that a double dose of beet supplementation every day for seven days before the target event produced a performance benefit.

You may wonder if you can juice your own beets to get the same benefits without having to take a supplement. You can, but unfortunately, it is difficult to know how many dietary nitrates you are actually consuming because of varying levels of nitrate concentration in the soil. On that note, it is important to research the company that produces the beet products you ingest, as some may not contain the amount of dietary nitrate needed for performance enhancement.

Also, be aware that a natural side effect of drinking beet juice is that your urine or feces changes to a pinkish-red color, but there is no reason to be alarmed. Beets are high in dietary oxalates as well. If you have a history of kidney stones, you may want to use caution with beet-juice supplementation.

Are Exogenous Ketones Helpful for Endurance Athletes?

The body usually uses three macronutrients—carbohydrates, fats, and proteins—for energy production. Ketones, or ketone bodies, are considered the fourth macronutrient and can be an alternative energy source, especially when energy from other sources is low. Ketone production typically occurs after bouts of fasting, extreme low-carbohydrate diets, and longer endurance exercise sessions.

In the early 2000s, the U.S. military became curious after research showed promise in ketones' ability to improve cognitive and physical performance in the field. In 2003, the Defense Advanced Research Projects Agency (DARPA) invested $10 million to develop a ketone ester product that could elevate blood ketone levels without going on a low-carbohydrate ketogenic diet (University of Oxford, 2016). In the years following the DARPA research, nutrition companies joined this trend. They started coming out with marketing-based ketone products such as raspberry ketones and ketone salt, supplements that have little to no impact on blood ketone levels. It wasn't until 2016, when Richard Veech and Kieran Clarke (the leaders of the DARPA research) released a ketone ester combined with alcohol, that exogenous ketone supplements started to show potential performance and recovery benefits (Cox et al. 2016). Interest really started booming within the endurance community when professional cycling teams started using them.

Possible Benefits

Research on exogenous ketone use in endurance athletes at this time is limited. Potential benefits of exogenous ketone use: includes a glycogen sparing effect, increased performance, mental alertness, and decreased recovery time.

- *Glycogen-sparing effect:* A proposed positive effect of exogenous ketone supplementation is the glycogen-sparing effect, which reduces the carbohydrates used during exercise and prolongs glycogen stores. In other words, you can keep gas in your gas tank for a longer time so that your high-quality fuel keeps you going at a higher effort for as long as possible, keeping muscle fatigue at bay. However, exogenous ketone supplementation has also been shown to reduce the body's ability to produce energy from carbohydrate sources at high-intensity efforts of 10 to 30 minutes, leaving athletes struggling to perform as well as they are capable.

- *Increased power:* Despite the mixed performance results using exogenous ketones alone, a 2021 study showed a 5 percent increase in power after three hours of exercise when consuming both exogenous ketones and sodium bicarbonate, a supplement used to buffer lactic acid during exercise (Poffé et al. 2021). Researchers theorize that this may be the result of sodium bicarbonate counteracting the acidosis produced by ketone consumption, unlocking the potential for ketones to benefit performance and giving athletes a boost.

- *Increased mental alertness:* In long events or races that go through the night, ketones might give competitors an edge by increasing alertness. Exogenous ketone supplements have been proposed as an option for maintaining mental acuity because of their effect on dopamine production. Higher dopamine concentration is associated with higher levels of energy and focus. One study of 18 recreational runners showed a significant increase in dopamine concentration during an 80K or 100K run, indicating a potential use for ketone supplements in events that require more mental acuity, such as trail and ultra-endurance runs (Poffé et al. 2023).

- *Postexercise recovery:* Increases in glycogen resynthesis and muscle protein synthesis rates after exercise have been observed when taking exogenous ketones with protein- and carbohydrate-rich fueling options (a postworkout smoothie or yogurt with granola). Quicker recovery of glycogen stores and muscle health could help athletes decrease muscle soreness, avoid injury, and return quicker for future training sessions.

- *Prevention of nonfunctional overreaching:* Some research has indicated that exogenous ketone supplementation helps prevent nonfunctional overreaching. Nonfunctional overreaching and overtraining syndrome are complex, poorly understood responses due to hormonal, nervous system, and energy dysregulation. This overlap of systems and symptoms makes it challenging to study, but results have indicated that ketones might help athletes adapt to training without overreaching. One study using daily exogenous ketone supplements inhibited overreaching symptoms, increased appetite (normally, appetite is decreased in over-reaching and overtraining states), and stimulated exercise adaptations (Poffé et al. 2019).While this study is promising, more research is needed to fully understand exogenous ketone supplementation and its impact on overreaching before it can be expertly recommended.

How to Supplement

Exogenous ketone supplements are sold as liquids made up of different chemical forms: ketone salt (beta-hydroxybutyric acid bound to sodium, magnesium, potassium, or calcium), alcoholic ketone (R-1,3-butanediol), and ketone ester (beta-hydroxybutyrate plus R-1,3-butanediol with an oxygen or ester bond).

While you can purchase exogenous ketones in different formulations, not all consumer products are created equal, and athletes should pay close attention. According to recent research by Evans et al. (2022), the salt and alcoholic forms may not raise blood ketone levels enough to effectively get the body into a ketogenic state. In other words, the salt and alcoholic forms may not be as effective. Based on these results, it would be best to supplement with ketone ester if you want to use exogenous ketones.

Potential Downsides

One of the challenges of ketone supplements is their foul taste, which some liken to cough syrup or straight alcohol, making them hard to consume, especially during exercise. To combat this issue, some companies try mixing ketones with a little bit of fruit flavor, but regardless, the taste is still distinct.

Other concerns include the potential for the supplements to cause upper and lower gastrointestinal symptoms like nausea, vomiting, cramping, and diarrhea.

A 2019 study had male and female participants use ketone monoesters and ketone salts and examined their gastrointestinal symptoms; ketone monoester products generated similar amounts of upper and lower gastrointestinal symptoms, while ketone salts tended to produce more upper gastrointestinal issues (Stubbs et al. 2019). Since taste preferences and gastrointestinal systems vary, proceed with caution. Make sure you try any ketone you plan on using in competition during training first.

The Bottom Line for Exogenous Ketones

While more research is underway, at the time of this book's publishing, the scope and scale of studies is limited. While ketones have attracted considerable attention in endurance sports, experts in the space recommend caution. While the future looks promising, the best available evidence right now indicates that focusing on less marginal nutritional gains is a better use of many athletes' time and energy.

Takeaways

- Endurance athletes should approach supplementation with nuance.
- While it is always preferred to get micronutrients from food, low levels of specific micronutrients such as iron, vitamin D, and magnesium could negatively impact an athlete's health and performance.
- Before supplementing, athletes should consider if dietary changes could get them to optimal levels, but some endurance athletes may find it difficult due to dietary preferences, lifestyle, or training.
- For possible ergogenic aids such as caffeine and ketones, athletes should ensure that the possible benefits outweigh the risks; if they choose to use said supplements, they should consider proper dosing and certified brands.
- While it may be tempting to immediately try supplementation, all other options to support health and performance goals should be considered first.

DESIGNING YOUR ADAPTABLE FUELING PLAN

I think the biggest thing that I have done nutritionwise that has contributed to my success is never to be completely satisfied with my fueling plan. I am constantly taking notes after big workouts and key sessions, tracking how I felt, environmental conditions, and any quantitative measures that might have stood out. My fueling strategy is always a work in progress. I feel like I need to have a plan for the conditions I'll be facing on race day and not just an overall plan that I aim to execute each race.

—Matt Hanson, professional triathlete and exercise scientist (athlete interview, 2022)

Picture this: You've trained for hours upon hours for a big upcoming race, and you think you have a fueling plan that will work. You throw together some calorie sources and plan to take only fluids on the course. Race day arrives, and it's extra hot and humid. You make it to the finish line, but just barely. Your stomach revolted, you had to make multiple pit stops, and you ended up in the med tent with dehydration after the race. What went wrong? You had nutrition and hydration during the race, but why didn't it work?

Having a baseline fueling plan is of utmost importance as an endurance athlete, but without the foresight to adjust your fueling plan to the environment, you could be setting yourself up for failure. Here enters the evolution of your fueling plan. If you are going to make it through an event successfully, you must consider the individual sport challenges, the potential environmental challenges, and the adjustments you may need to make as an endurance athlete if something goes wrong.

When something goes awry during a race or adventure, many endurance athletes like to blame their food or calorie choices as the main cause of their issues. Unfortunately, this view tends to neglect hydration and electrolyte intake, two other keys to a successful fueling plan. To have a working fueling plan, fluid, electrolyte, and calorie intake should all be carefully analyzed and personalized to your individual requirements months in advance of a target event. General recommendations are often given for these keys, but they are not the most accurate way to build and test the plan.

Your fueling plan should be an adjustable framework based on your training and racing goals. If you are competing in multiple endurance sports, you will need to make the necessary and practical adjustments to ensure everything is properly optimized.

Sweat Rate and Fluid Consumption

When determining appropriate fluid intake for your workout or race, you need to factor in your sweat rate. Sweat production is an essential physiological process that helps maintain body temperature during exercise. The body's core temperature rises during exercise, particularly during higher intensities and when exposed to different environmental conditions (e.g., hot temperatures and humidity). Sweat is produced in special glands dispersed throughout the body; when it evaporates on the skin, it releases heat (Baker 2017).

Sweat composition is highly individual, but it contains predominantly sodium, chloride, magnesium, calcium, and phosphorus. Sodium, found in its largest quantities in our intracellular space, is the electrolyte lost in the highest amounts through sweat and has the biggest impact on total body hydration status (Montain and Coyle 1992). When trying to determine fluid and electrolyte requirements during exercise, focus on sweat sodium concentration test results.

Everyone has their own fluid loss rates, which will determine target replenishment rates during exercise. Sweat fluid loss rates can change depending on several factors such as your genetic predisposition, number of sweat glands, body weight, metabolism, and fitness level. Sweat sodium concentration is not nearly as variable. It is well known that excessive fluid loss of more than 2 percent of body weight can impact performance, so minimizing sodium loss is key (Sawka et al. 2007).

For training and events lasting one to two hours, thirst is a reasonable way to determine how much fluid to consume. However, for longer bouts of exercise, it is important to account for fluid losses and plan intake more precisely. Because fluid loss rates can change, regularly testing fluid loss (ideally quarterly) can help you determine fluid replenishment rates more precisely.

Calculating Fluid Loss Rates

You can estimate your personal fluid loss rates fairly easily by following these steps:

1. Weigh yourself naked before a low-intensity hour-long training session.
2. Weigh yourself naked after the low-intensity training session.
3. Subtract your weight after the session from your weight before the session to determine, in ounces or milliliters, how much fluid you lost during exercise.
4. Add the number of ounces or milliliters of fluids you consumed during the training session.
5. Repeat this process at least two more times (on different days) and take the average of all three to get your average fluid loss during low-intensity training sessions.
6. Once you have an average, aim to take in 75 to 90 percent of your average fluid loss during every hour of activity, leaving room for error.

For example, if you find you lose 1 pound (16 ounces or 480 milliliters) on average during a one-hour training session, 75 to 90 percent is 12 to 14.4 ounces (360 to 432 milliliters), which would be your fluid intake goal every hour.

If you find that you lose more than 34 ounces of fluid (about 1 liter) per hour, your strategy should be adjusted, as it can be logistically difficult to consume that much fluid every hour. In addition, the gut's absorptive capacity is limited, so it may not be possible to consume that much fluid each hour, in which case reducing the gravity of the fluid deficit becomes the main goal.

Sodium Concentration Testing

Unlike fluid loss, which changes under different conditions, sweat sodium concentration is relatively genetic. This can be quite beneficial for athletes because if you choose to have your sweat sodium concentration evaluated, you likely won't need to keep testing it. Slight variations can occur because of the amount of sodium in the diet and heat acclimatization protocols, but this can be hard to fully quantify. Since sweat sodium concentration varies slightly, its replenishment rate should match the fluid loss rate: consume 75 to 90 percent of the loss every hour. Think of your sweat sodium concentration as a marker to put you into one of three boxes—low sodium sweater, medium sodium sweater, or high sodium sweater—and work from there.

In an ideal world, everyone would use the whole-body washdown sweat collection method to figure out sweat sodium loss because it's the most accurate, but unfortunately, it's usually not practical for the everyday endurance athlete. The following are all methods currently on the market for testing your sweat sodium concentration:

- *Whole-body washdown:* The body is washed down after exercise, the sweat is analyzed, and the results give a picture of full-body sweat losses without interrupting the normal sweat process. While this is the most accurate method of sweat sodium testing, it is very impractical because it must be done in a lab and often doesn't reflect real-life sport conditions.

- *Sweat patches:* An absorbable patch is applied to the skin and picks up sweat. The patch is then placed in a sealed tube and sent off to a lab for analysis. A downside of the patch is that it can cover sweat glands and block them from functioning normally.

Calculating Your Fluid Loss Rate and Sweat Sodium Concentration

Use your fluid loss rate and sweat sodium concentration to formulate your winning fluid and electrolyte replenishment strategy:

1. Take average fluid loss rate per hour and multiply by 0.75 and 0.90 to get a target replenishment range for every hour of exercise.

2. Once your target fluid replenishment rate has been established, multiply your sweat sodium concentration by your fluid replenishment rate to get your target sodium replenishment rate.

Use the following example as a guide:

Fluid loss rate = 32 oz/hr

To get your target fluid intake range, do the following:

32 oz × 0.75 = 24 oz

32 oz × 0.90 = 29 oz

Target fluid intake range per hour = 24-29 oz

Sweat sodium concentration = 44 mg/oz

To get your target sodium intake range, do the following:

44 mg × 24 oz = 1,056 mg

44 mg × 29 oz = 1,246 mg

Target sodium intake range per hour = 1,056-1,246 mg

Upset Stomach and Fueling Plan Adjustments

If your stomach decides to revolt during exercise, it can be difficult to figure out what to do next. While it may be tempting to completely avoid taking in calories or fluids, this may only exacerbate your symptoms. Here are some tips on how to continue fueling despite an upset stomach:

1. *Try to continue taking in calories:* Use liquid calories if you can still stomach something like a hydration mix.

2. *Mix it up with savory:* After a longer period of taking in sweet items, the body can be overcome with palate fatigue. Having savory options available, such as mashed potatoes or pretzels, may be the perfect reset your system needs.

3. *Carry Tums, peppermints, or ginger chews:* While these options may be temporary solutions to a bigger problem, they can allow your stomach to settle just enough to try to get nutrition in.

4. *Suck on candy or chews:* Sucking on candy or chews can let a slight drip of nutrition into the body when nothing else will work.

- *Biometric sweat-testing devices (wearables):* These devices use technology to sense fluid and electrolyte losses, and they analyze and transmit the data to an app for real-time results. The accuracy of many of these wearables has not been validated by scientific research, which makes them a somewhat unreliable method for figuring out sodium loss.

Sweat sodium concentration loss is typically expressed as milligrams per liter of sweat. For ease of use in a fueling plan, I usually standardize the concentration to milligrams of sodium lost per ounce or milliliter of sweat. This allows athletes to match their sodium concentration to their target fluid intake when building a fueling plan. To get your sweat sodium concentration in milligrams per ounce, divide the milligrams per liter by 33.8 ounces. Once both fluid loss and sodium concentration are measured, they can be combined to design the perfect fueling plan.

How to Fuel in Extreme Environments

In 2016, Jax Mariash Mustafa, aptly named the "queen of the desert," became the first female in race history to finish the 4 Deserts Grand Slam Plus, a series of multiday running races in some of the most extreme environments in the world. The challenge consists of the Roving Race plus the 4 Deserts Race in the hottest (Namibia), windiest (Gobi March), driest (Atacama Crossing), and coldest (Antarctica) deserts in the world.

Her experiences in these races required a specific set of physical and mental training techniques that allowed her to reach the finish lines healthy and in one piece. She often ran out of water before the next aid station, but she had trained her mind to keep going by taking "air sips" out of her bottle just to make it to the next checkpoint. This took a lot of mental strength.

Physically, trying to stay cool with the smallest amount of water on key sweat points allowed her core body temperature to stay down, even when the outside temperature was well over 135 degrees Fahrenheit at times. She used sauna and heat bath protocols before the events so her body could adapt to extremes before she arrived for the races.

Calculating her fluid and electrolyte losses ahead of time allowed her to know that she would need at least three bottles of water with extra electrolytes every hour to withstand the conditions. Testing the melting and freezing points of food options let her choose fuel that would withstand the various extremes. Prior to competing in these races, Jax tried to get by with as little nutrition as possible to help her learn to withstand the extreme conditions.

For endurance athletes considering training or racing in extreme conditions, specific personalized approaches are a must in order to perform. The rest of this chapter will help you understand how best to practice your fueling and hydration intake if you plan to train or race under these conditions.

Altitude

When it comes to getting high—that is, higher altitude—endurance athletes who train at high altitudes to gain performance benefits need to consider the impacts this has on their nutritional requirements. There is no consensus in the running community about how much resting metabolic rate (RMR) changes at high altitudes; however, there does seem to be a threefold increase of RMR at higher altitudes (Butterfield et al. 1992). Endurance athletes training and racing at extremely high altitudes need to be aware of these increases and plan accordingly to meet increased intake needs with nutrient-dense foods. Even at moderately high altitudes, energy requirements may increase, but the extent to which that increase occurs and how long it remains elevated is not conclusively known.

Macronutrient Requirements

While overall energy requirements increase with altitude, macronutrient shifts should be considered to account for side effects of hypoxia.

Carbohydrates

At higher altitudes, the preferred macronutrients for energy production are carbohydrates because they require 10 percent less oxygen to produce energy compared to fats and proteins. Taking in appropriate carbohydrate amounts is important to replenish glycogen stores and prevent muscle protein breakdown as well as prevent high-altitude mountain sickness, dizziness, and vomiting. Choosing simple carbohydrates such as juice, white rice, or tortillas over more complex sources may be most helpful if you lose your appetite.

Proteins

Extreme high altitude has been shown to lead to increased muscle wasting. It is important to focus on getting adequate carbohydrate (protein-sparing) and protein amounts in regular daily intervals to maximize muscle protein synthesis rates. BCAA supplements (leucine, isoleucine, and valine) may also be beneficial at higher altitudes because of their propensity to promote the highest rates of muscle protein synthesis.

Fats

Fats, while nutrient dense, are not the preferred fuel at high altitude because they require higher oxygen amounts to produce energy. However, consuming some fats is important for maintaining overall energy intake and maximizing fat-soluble vitamin absorption.

A Note on Appetite Suppression

At high altitude, the body alters the hormones leptin and cholecystokinin, which promote fullness, and this can make it harder for athletes to fuel themselves appropriately. Digestive enzyme production and gastric motility may also decrease, causing malabsorption and a feeling of fullness. Strategies to combat appetite loss include consuming more liquid calorie options (smoothies and soups), food blends (fruit blends, applesauce, and mashed potatoes), nut and seed butters (peanut butter, cashew butter, almond butter, and pumpkin seed butter), and energy-dense cookies and pastries.

Vanilla Butterfly Pea Tea Recovery Smoothie

This uniquely flavored smoothie packs in a lot of carbohydrates and protein to replenish your glycogen stores and repair muscles, especially when you lack an appetite.

Servings: 1

Ingredients

- 1 cup (160 g) frozen banana
- 1 cup (240 mL) milk or milk alternative
- 1 cup (230 g or 240 mL) frozen oranges or orange juice
- 1/4 tsp vanilla extract or paste
- 1 scoop vanilla protein powder
- 1 tsp butterfly pea tea powder
- 1/4 avocado for extra fat, protein, and creaminess if desired

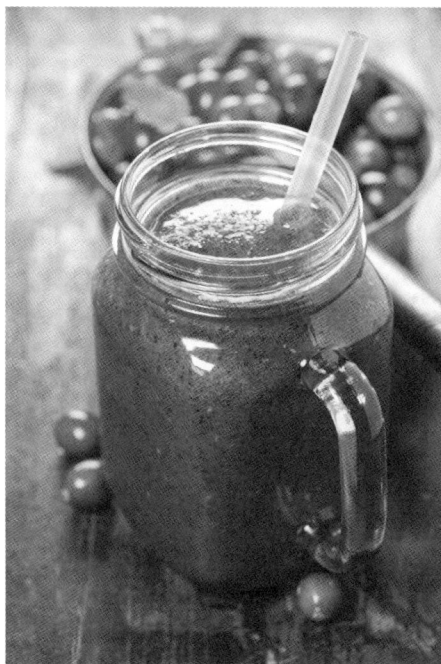

Directions

Add to a blender and puree until smooth and creamy.

Professional Chef/Sports Nutrition.

The Picture Pantry/Alloy/Getty Images

Micronutrients

At high altitude, oxidative stress increases and can increase free radical production in the body, which negatively affects performance and recovery time. Supplementation with the antioxidants vitamin C, vitamin E, selenium, and zinc can help fight cellular damage caused by oxidative stressors.

Arguably, the most important micronutrient of concern at high altitude is iron because of its important role in oxygen use in the body. A dose-dependent response occurs with iron supplementation at high altitude. In 2015, Govus et al. demonstrated that athletes who went to training camps at high altitudes and didn't supplement iron experienced much lower increases in hemoglobin (1.2 percent), while those who did supplement with 105 milligrams and 210 milligrams of iron experienced hemoglobin increases of 3.3 percent and 4 percent, respectively. This is of particular importance due to hemoglobin's role as a vital link between oxygen availability and energy production. It is important that endurance athletes have a good understanding of their blood iron levels before going to high altitudes and deciding to supplement. Be sure to test your blood iron levels before supplementing to avoid risking iron overload, digestive upset, and inhibited absorption of other micronutrients that compete with iron at absorption sites.

Hydration

At higher elevations, hydration requirements are higher due to increases in fluid lost in respiration (lower amounts of oxygen cause an increase in respiration rate). Fluid needs may be increased up to 1.5 times the normal requirements. To stay hydrated, endurance athletes should develop an altitude-specific hydration protocol that includes water-rich fruits and vegetables, sports drinks, and herbal teas.

Nutrition Checklist for Training and Racing at High Altitude

1. Have a full iron panel done at least four to six weeks before traveling to an area of high altitude. If ferritin levels fall below 40 to 50 milligrams per milliliter, iron supplementation every day can be considered.

2. Be prepared for a decrease in appetite and an increase in energy requirements. Plan easy-to-consume, energy-dense, carbohydrate-rich snacks and meals, including liquid options such as smoothies and juices.

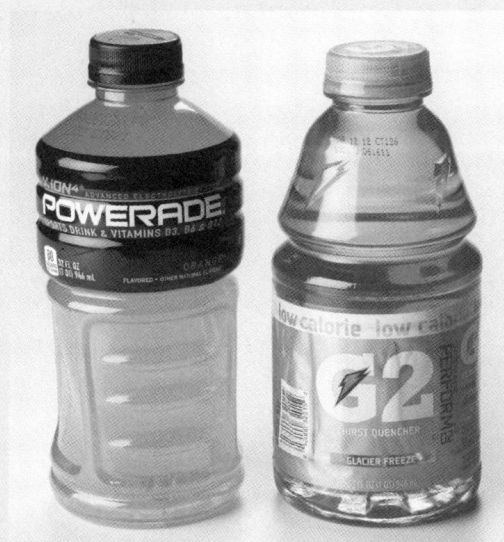

Electrolyte drinks can help with recovery and increase your whole body's hydration.

3. Increased respiratory water loss and lower humidity will cause an increased risk of dehydration. Be proactive by monitoring urine color and being aware of thirst to stay on top of hydration. Taking in an electrolyte supplement with fluids can increase your whole body's hydration.

4. Be prepared for sleep disturbances. Higher altitudes can cause initial sleep disturbances due to hypoxic conditions. Stay hydrated and try to stick to normal sleep routines to support your circadian rhythm.

Heat and Humidity

Endurance exercise in the heat and humidity has its own unique challenges when it comes to fueling. Hot and humid conditions can cause the cardiorespiratory, thermoregulatory, and gastrointestinal systems to become dysregulated, putting health and performance at risk. Being able to adapt to hot and humid environments with specific fueling strategies can help you successfully train and race in these conditions.

During exercise, the body produces heat as a by-product of muscle contraction and loses heat through the skin as it sweats. This process is controlled by neural thermoreceptors in the skin, but the body's internal temperature can rise if it is not able to rid itself of heat fast enough because of clothing, sunlight exposure, wind exposure, or the intensity, duration, or type of exercise. Heavier, nonbreathable clothing provides a barrier that prevents heat loss. Choosing looser, breathable clothing that is lighter in color can dissipate heat. While direct sunlight increases internal body temperature, wind can cool the body by exacerbating heat loss from the skin. According to a 2019 review by Bouscaren, Millet, and Racinais, exercise intensity is the main factor in heat production, with higher intensity leading to more heat.

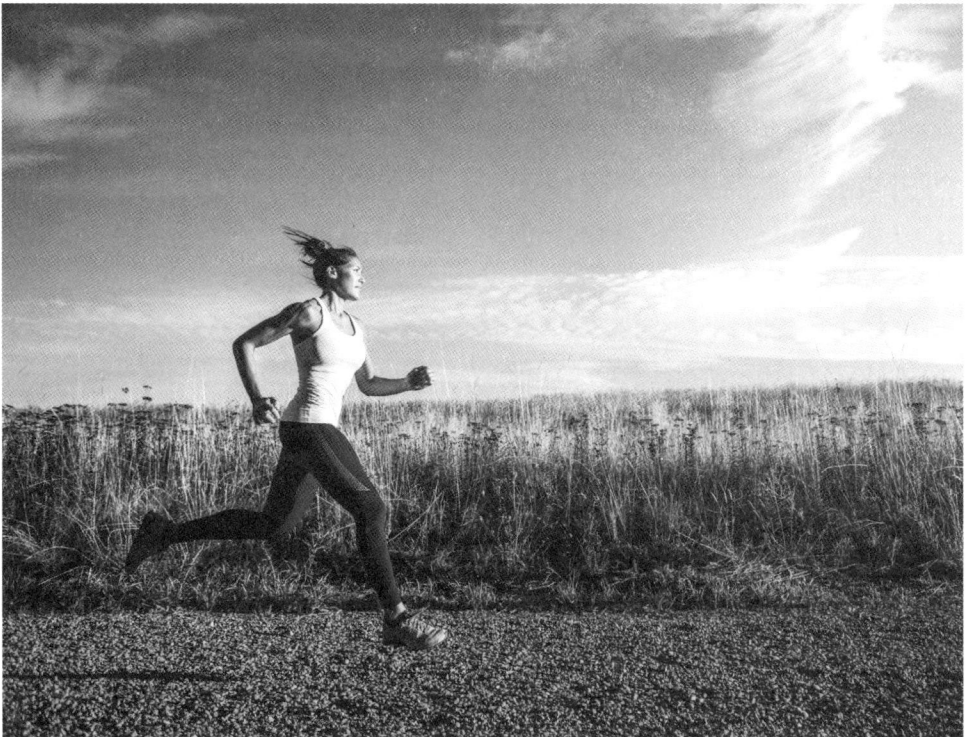

RyanJLane/Getty Images

Athletes can employ heat acclimation or heat acclimatization in their training to prepare their body for performing in events in heat and humidity.

High heat exposure during exercise can compromise the gastrointestinal tract's function and permeability more than normal. During exercise, blood is diverted away from the gastrointestinal system, and overall digestive capacity is reduced. This can result in mucosal lining degradation, reduced gastric emptying, reduced nutrient absorption, and hyperpermeability of the cells that make up the intestinal lining.

To mitigate the negative effects of heat and humidity on the body, endurance athletes can employ heat acclimation, heat acclimatization, and specific nutrition strategies. Heat acclimation involves repeatedly exposing the body to heat stress for 7 to 14 days through tools such as hot baths and saunas. This allows the body to adapt by reducing heart rate, improving sodium resorption, and improving fluid balance control. Heat acclimatization involves traveling to a particular climate and living there for a period of time to let the body adjust.

Regarding nutrition, fluid and electrolyte consumption before, during, and after a workout appear to have the biggest impact on heat and humidity tolerance. Endurance athletes need to avoid the 2 percent body fluid loss by preparing a working fluid and electrolyte strategy to reduce strain on the cardiorespiratory system and prevent performance impairment.

Hydration and Electrolyte Strategies Before Exercise

Endurance athletes working in hot and humid conditions need to monitor their hydration status. Starting in a dehydrated state reduces an athlete's ability to tolerate heat and perform well.

Ingesting fluids containing electrolytes (particularly sodium) can help you retain fluid and avoid hyponatremia (low blood sodium with an imbalance between total body water and electrolytes). Sodium solutions taken before exercise can also increase blood plasma volume and better maintain that volume during exercise. While consuming a higher concentration of sodium in the two hours before exercise can help you hydrate, too much (over 4,000 milligrams per liter) can lead to gastrointestinal distress. According to the ACSM consensus statement from 2007, consuming 500 milliliters of fluids two hours before exercise gives it enough time for to properly assimilate into the body (Sawka et al.).

Preloading with sodium in the days before an event may not be necessary, but it can be helpful to sip on and electrolyte solution starting one to three days before race day to avoid hyponatremia.

Consider the temperature of fluids you consume before exercise in hot environments; consuming ice slurry beverages (plain ice slurry, crushed ice, or sports drink ice slurry) 30 minutes before exercising may help your core body temperature stay lower and preserve gastrointestinal integrity. Combining an ice slurry with a menthol mouth rinse can expand heat regulation time and has been shown to extend running performance time in heat and humidity (Gopathi, Tiwari, and Kalpana 2023).

Hydration and Electrolyte Strategies During Exercise

The scientific community debates whether planned or drinking-to-thirst strategies are best for fluid replacement during exercise; however, what is not debated is that more than a 2 percent loss in body fluids can lead to performance reductions. Heat increases fluid loss as the body tries to cool down the system to maintain internal temperature. Fluid replenishment relying on thirst alone in high heat may become difficult the longer the event and the more extreme the temperatures. Keeping fluids cooler (less than 70 degrees Fahrenheit), if possible to obtain or carry during exercise, has been shown to increase palatability and consumption. Sodium consumption during exercise may help maintain fluid balance and reduce the risk of hyponatremia, but there is no consensus on how much sodium to take in during exercise. Sweat sodium concentration and fluid loss testing can help an endurance athlete personalize their fluid and electrolyte plan and develop strategies for planned intake.

Hydration and Electrolyte Strategies After Exercise

Replenishment of lost fluids after exercise should equal 150 percent of the fluids lost. Consuming fluids with food can help you absorb the fluids and hydrate fully. Replenishing sodium immediately after exercise may help you retain fluid and your body come back into balance. Using concentrated electrolyte supplements that contain a mix of sodium, potassium, magnesium, chloride, and calcium can help with the process, or simply salting food with extra table salt can help too (1/4 teaspoon of table salt contains about 575 milligrams of sodium). Continue to replenish fluids and electrolytes for the rest of the day until the loss gaps are closed.

Strategies for Reducing Gastrointestinal Distress

Heat places increased stress on the gastrointestinal tract, so it is important to consider nutrition strategies to reduce this stress in the heat.

- Before competition, consider eating carbohydrates with lower fiber as well as smaller amounts of proteins and fats.
- Fermentable oligosaccharides, disaccharides, monosaccharides, and polyols (FODMAP) are carbohydrates that may be harder for some athletes to digest and absorb in the small intestine (e.g., fruit, gluten-containing grains, dairy, and some nuts). Avoiding individual offenders may help you avoid stomach distress. It is important for endurance athletes to remember that engaging in a low-FODMAP diet should always be a temporary elimination diet to help figure out which FODMAP-containing foods are problematic. See more details on this diet in chapter 6.

- A fueling strategy that includes consuming frequent but small amounts of carbohydrates instead of large amounts of carbohydrates can allow for more effective absorption.

- Be mindful of carbohydrate sources during exercise; reliance on carbohydrates from fluids may become problematic if you are unable to consume unpalatable solutions.

Troubleshooting Muscle Cramping

The cause of and solution for exercise-associated muscle cramps (EAMC) is complex; this multifaceted issue can be highly frustrating for endurance athletes to navigate. Painful and spasmodic cramps during training and racing can interfere with or ruin an athlete's performance. EAMC can range from light cramps to full-body spasms and can last a few minutes or longer. Unfortunately, they tend to be very unpredictable, and some athletes appear to be more susceptible to them.

Studies have attempted to figure out correlated causes of muscle cramps, but because they are hard to induce or predict, it's hard to study them and identify causes. Some hypotheses for muscle cramping include water and electrolyte imbalances, dysregulated muscle motor complex, low carbohydrate availability, and lack of training adaptations to the proposed exercise (Maughan and Shirreffs 2019).

1. *Water and electrolyte imbalances:* Some studies have looked at the relationship between total fluid and electrolyte losses and muscle cramping. While larger losses have been associated with a higher risk of cramping, the mechanism and pattern is not clearly understood.

2. *Dysregulated muscle motor complex:* This idea proposes that muscle cramping is caused by an abnormality of alpha neuron control at the spinal level but does not have an underlying explanation for the cause of said abnormality.

3. *Low carbohydrate availability:* Because carbohydrates have an impact on overall energy production and muscle fatigue levels, not fueling with enough carbohydrates can lead to increased muscular fatigue levels, which is associated with an increased risk of muscle cramps.

4. *Lack of training adaptations:* High intensity, long duration, hilly terrain, or higher altitude that an endurance athlete has not trained for enough can contribute to muscle fatigue. Training adaptations allow athletes to expand plasma volume and develop neuromuscular fatigue resistance, which can help prevent muscle cramping.

Overall, EAMC is a complex topic that can affect the body's ability to turn off muscle contractions, leaving them turned on or stuck. By identifying all possible causes of EAMC, an endurance athlete can reduce their risk of developing muscle cramps with the understanding that fully preventing them may not be possible.

Cold

Just as with heat, training and racing in cold temperatures requires its own set of unique recommendations. Fueling choices that work well in the heat may freeze at lower temperatures; hydration becomes more of a challenge because the risk of fluids freezing is much higher.

As we consider cold-weather training and racing, let's break down the components of any fueling plan and focus on what might be of particular concern to endurance athletes.

Fluids

Because fluids keep the body operating properly in many ways, and we know that even slight dehydration can affect performance, we need to carefully monitor our fluids, even on the coldest of days. Fluid loss rates will still vary depending on the athlete, which is why regular fluid loss testing is very important for athletes.

Winter-Specific Tips

When training in the winter, the body experiences cold weather diuresis, reacting to cold temperatures to avoid hypothermia by keeping blood close to the organs and away from the extremities and skin. This can increase blood pressure, which causes the body to feel the need to urinate frequently. Thirst response can also become blunted. This does not mean that your body is properly hydrated and that you should skip the fluids. You are still sweating and losing fluids during winter training. Clothing choices and respiration in general also contribute to overall fluid loss.

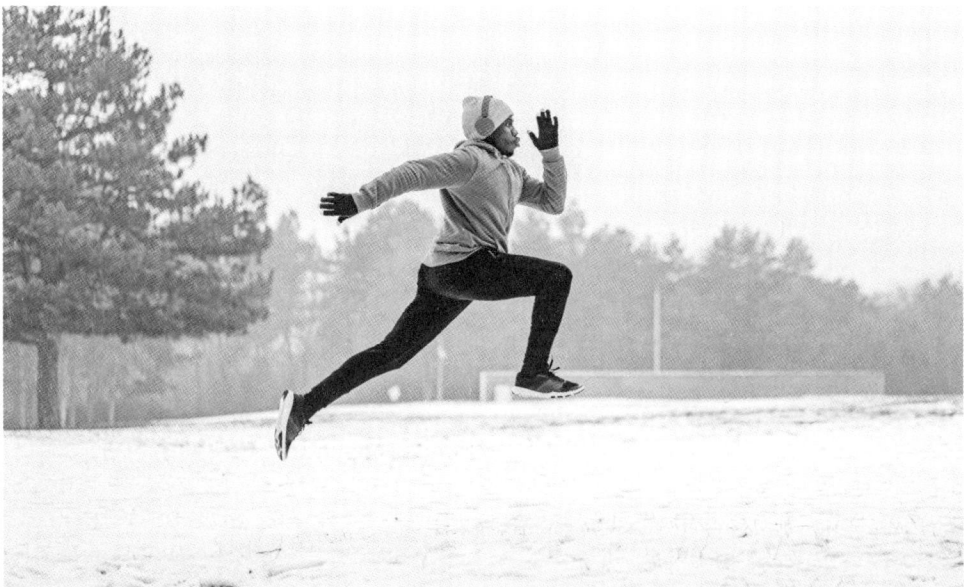

urbazon/E+/Getty Images

To reduce fluid losses, make sensible clothing choices when training and participating in cold climates.

Because of these factors, cold temperatures usually require an athlete to have a more targeted fluid intake strategy rather than relying on thirst signals. Having an intake target every hour, with reminders or alarms, may help you consume enough.

Practical Tips
Preventing fluids from freezing is key to a strategic plan. Strategies include the following:

- Use an insulated bladder hose.
- Wrap your bottles in wool socks or other insulation materials or create a front pouch to keep your fluids closer to the center of your body.
- Blow into water bottle caps and hoses after consuming fluids to prevent complete freezing, which would leave you unable to obtain fluids.
- Put hot water in your bottles to start out with warmer liquids.
- Weigh the pluses and minuses of getting calories from liquids. For example, it could help skiers who have a hard time chewing their fuel due to pole logistics, but if the fluids freeze and they don't have a backup plan, it could be disastrous.

Sodium and Electrolyte Intake

Sodium is the most important when it comes to electrolytes lost in sweat, and you may or may not need to replace those electrolytes during winter activities because your fluid loss rates are probably lower.

Winter-Specific Considerations
Knowing your sweat sodium concentration and your fluid loss rates can be important when you're trying to figure out if and how much you need to replace in the winter. For longer ski mountaineering, Nordic skiing, or touring events, it may be wise to calculate sodium needs to avoid hyponatremia. Keep in mind that at high altitudes, electrolyte needs may be higher. Because of the extremely cold temperatures you may exercise in, it is important to have separate fueling and gear strategies to tackle the challenges you might face in these conditions.

Calories and Carbohydrates

Carbohydrates act as your fuel during activity. Remember that stored carbohydrate (glycogen) will give you about 90 minutes to 2 hours of endurance activity without too much fatigue. Once your glycogen stores are emptied, your body will make energy from fat stores and muscle protein breakdown, but it is a less efficient process and will likely leave you feeling more fatigued.

Calorie and carbohydrate consumption during exercise typically comes from a variety of sources. Remember that relying predominantly on

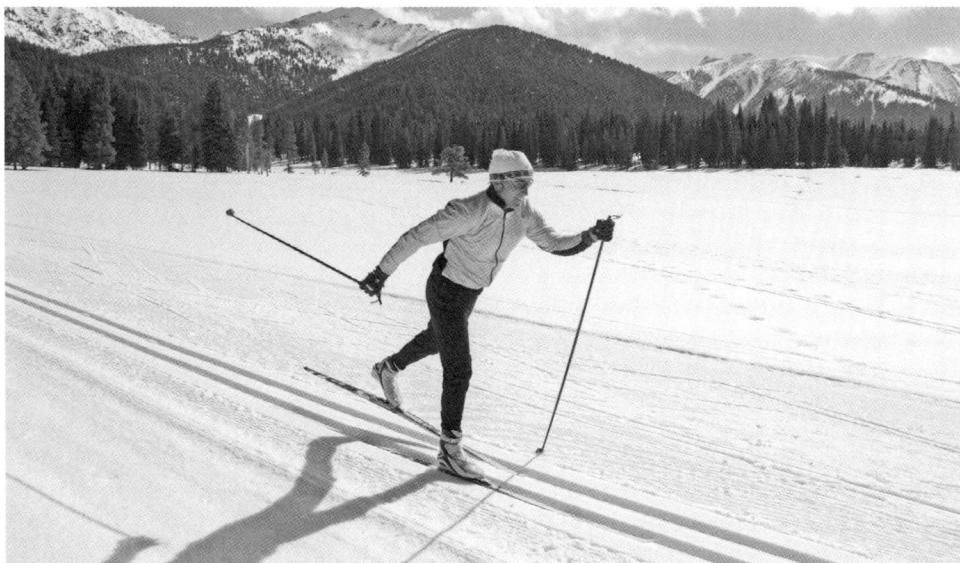

For skiing or touring events, it is wise to choose fuel sources wisely and hold them close to the body to prevent freezing.

fluids for fuel in the winter can have detrimental effects if they freeze. You may need to do some testing to see what will work because gels and chews you use in the heat may not work in the cold.

Practical Tips

When considering fuel options for winter endurance sports, use the following ideas to figure out your options before going to the backcountry or trails.

- Hold your gels and chews close to your body.
- Put fuel choices in the freezer to see how they respond to cold temperatures.
- Whole-food options may work better during cold months. These include muffins, food blends, and cookies. Consider the portability and practicality of these foods when making your choices, and be sure to practice your fueling plan beforehand.

Takeaways

- Your baseline fueling plan should be a blueprint to support your training and performance goals. It should be adaptable to account for your sport and the upcoming event duration, terrain, and environmental conditions.
- Take the time to get curious and figure out your sweat sodium loss and fluid loss, and experiment with different calorie-containing modalities. This will help you learn to pivot and become an adaptable athlete when conditions are unpredictable. Who knows? It just might save your race.

4

CONSIDERATIONS FOR THE FEMALE ATHLETE

One of the single most important things I have learned as a female elite endurance athlete is the importance of using my period as an indicator light for myself. I've never missed one but made a conscious effort to learn how to fuel myself as uniquely female. I have learned how to navigate racing and fueling with my period and during this transition into perimenopause. I want there to be more conversation in this space and hope that other endurance athletes can celebrate and optimize being female, finding what works with their unique bodies, not against [them].

—Camille Herron, professional ultra runner and female 100-mile world record holder

While foundational nutrition recommendations and skills remain constant regardless of gender, more and more research is emerging about the individual physiology of female athletes and the hormonal factors that affect women and their nutritional requirements throughout different phases of life (from menses to postmenopause). Regarding micronutrient and macronutrient requirements and nutrition timing, female endurance athletes are hungry for a more personalized approach. Until the last decade, endurance sports nutrition research was predominantly focused on male endurance athletes. This complicates things because with limited research available, data can be extrapolated to support the most desirable ideas. This chapter will focus on what we do know and how women can best work with their physiology to optimize endurance performance.

Menstrual Cycle

Let's be clear. Our periods should be celebrated, not feared or shunned. Unfortunately, in the endurance sports space, athletes can get this message: "Well, you're an endurance athlete, so not getting your period is normal." The reality is that your period is an indicator light and should be treated as one. While things such as birth control can affect your monthly cycle, regularly skipping periods is not normal and can have detrimental consequences for future bone health and performance.

As a refresher, the average length of a menstrual cycle is between 26 and 28 days (this can vary, though) and can be divided into four main phases: menses, follicular, ovulation, and luteal. Menses begins the first day you start bleeding and can last from one to seven days. The follicular phase includes menses and usually lasts from days 1 to 16. Ovulation is the time in the cycle when an egg is released from the ovaries, and it lasts just 24 hours. The luteal phase includes ovulation and starts midway through the cycle (around day 14) after an egg is released from the ovaries. It is important to understand the four phases of the menstrual cycle because hormones fluctuate throughout.

Periods often come with symptoms, which many women worry will affect their performance. Premenstrual syndrome (PMS) symptoms can occur anytime in the luteal phase, but are most common in the seven days before menstruation begins. Some women experience symptoms such as depression, breast tenderness, irritability, fatigue, and bloating. Menstrual symptoms can also include cramping, bloating, upset stomach, mood swings, and sleep disruptions. All these symptoms can be mitigated by giving attention to proper nutrition throughout the month.

No Period: A Key Indicator for RED-S?

Lack of a monthly period may indicate that an athlete is struggling with LEA, which correlates with RED-S (see chapter 1 for more on this topic). To support regular, healthy cycles, young athletes should establish healthy fueling behaviors in high school and college.

What Impact Does a Female Athlete's Cycle Have on Performance?

Physiological changes occur throughout the menstrual cycle that affect endurance performance through muscle activation, body composition, temperature regulation, and energy utilization. While it appears that nutrition changes during the different phases of the cycle can influence performance, it is important to note that more research on nutrition for female athletes is needed. Here is what we know.

Estrogen, which is high during the follicular and late luteal phases, has an anabolic effect, improving muscle strength and bone density. During times of higher estrogen, this has a protein-sparing effect (muscle mass is preserved), and women have higher rates of lipid metabolism and lower rates of carbohydrate and protein metabolism compared to men (Holtzman and Ackerman 2021). In the follicular stage, protein can be emphasized, but in the luteal phase, which has a drop in estrogen, protein intake should increase because of higher rates of protein catabolism.

Macronutrient Requirements

Female endurance athletes should not fear carbohydrates. Your body uses and stores carbohydrates more rapidly in the follicular phase than in the luteal phase. In the first half of your cycle (follicular phase), aim for a preworkout meal or snack that contains one gram of carbohydrate per kilogram one to four hours before exercise to optimize carbohydrate availability. During exercise, carbohydrates are still best for energy production. Aim for a minimum of 30 to 60 grams of carbohydrate per hour; some athletes can tolerate up to 90 grams per hour. After exercise, glycogen replenishment rates will vary depending on which phase of your cycle you are in. Glycogen storage rates are slower in the follicular phase compared to the luteal phase, so emphasizing quick consumption of carbohydrates after high-intensity exercise and workouts longer than 90 minutes is particularly important during the first half of your cycle.

Fats are the building blocks of hormones, so having enough of them is crucial for maintaining a healthy cycle. Female endurance athletes use fats at a higher rate than their male counterparts, and overall fat oxidation (utilization) rates are higher in the second half of the cycle. Focusing on inclusion, not extreme restriction of fat sources in the diet, should be the focus of any endurance athlete to ensure a healthy, functioning female body.

It is of the utmost importance that female endurance athletes meet the energy demands of their sport. Well-controlled studies have shown that optimal energy intake for women to maintain psychological function is 45 kilocalories per kilogram of FFM per day (Mountjoy et al. 2018). Inadequate energy intake will have a bigger impact overall than any manipulation of macronutrients will because neglecting to meet energy demands can lead lost periods and decreased bone density (Mountjoy et al. 2018). Female endurance athletes exercising 6 to 10 hours per week need at least 2,500 calories or more per day; anything less risks macro- and micronutrient deficiencies. Throughout the menstrual cycle, daily energy needs may vary, with some studies showing that athletes need 2.5 to 11.5 percent more calories during the second half of their cycles (see table 4.1). Age also plays a role in dictating energy needs. For postmenopausal athletes, metabolism and energy needs may decrease because of declining muscle mass, which should be considered when estimating requirements (Mishra, Mishra, and Devanshi 2011).

Micronutrient Requirements

Micronutrient requirements for athletes who get a period can vary, but in general, they should focus on an increased need for the following:

• *Iron:* Iron losses are higher in menstruating female athletes due to monthly blood loss. Some symptoms of low iron include fatigue, brittle hair and nails, cold sensitivity, and trouble breathing. Menstruating endurance athletes should have annual iron panels to test TIBC, iron saturation percentage, serum iron, and ferritin levels.

• *Vitamin D:* Because of its role in aiding the absorption of calcium, which affects bone health, vitamin D is also a micronutrient of concern for female athletes. In a study that included 102 National College Athletic Association (NCAA) female athletes at a single college, more than 20 percent of them were found to be vitamin D deficient (Villacis et al. 2014). Because few foods contain vitamin D, supplementation may be necessary to reach daily needs.

• *Calcium:* Women need higher amounts of calcium from their diet to prevent bone stress injuries and osteoporosis development. Suggested intake is around 1,500 milligrams per day, and supplementation should be considered if needs cannot be met from the diet (Holtzman and Ackerman 2021).

If you are looking for a more practical way to implement these changes, the following is an example of a sample menu that accounts for varying nutrition needs throughout the menstrual cycle.

First Half of Cycle (Follicular Phase)
This plan adds extra carbohydrate to the preworkout snack to account for reduced glycogen storage during this phase of the cycle.

Breakfast: Two eggs, two pieces of toast, yogurt, berries

Lunch: Turkey sandwich with cheese, carrots with hummus, orange

Preworkout snack: Four graham crackers with honey, banana

Postworkout snack: Protein shake, two cookies, applesauce

Dinner: Three tofu tacos on corn tortillas with beans, lettuce, tomato, and onion

Snack: Cottage cheese with pineapple

Second Half of Cycle (Luteal Phase)
This plan is slightly higher in protein, fat, and calories to account for changes in fat and protein metabolism throughout the cycle.

Breakfast: Three eggs, two pieces of toast, yogurt, banana

Lunch: Turkey sandwich with cheese and avocado, carrots with hummus, orange, almonds

Preworkout snack: Three graham crackers with a little bit of nut butter

Postworkout snack: Protein shake, two cookies

Dinner: Three tofu tacos on corn tortillas with avocado, lettuce, tomato, and onion

Snack: Cottage cheese with pineapple, a few squares of dark chocolate

TABLE 4.1 Summary of Menstrual-Cycle-Specific Nutrition Changes

Phase of cycle	Calories	Protein	Carbohydrate	Fat	Micronutrients
Follicular (days 1-14): Estrogen and progesterone remain low.	Energy needs remain at baseline.	Protein oxidation (breakdown) decreases, which does not warrant any dietary changes.	Carbohydrate oxidation rates increase, and glycogen storage capabilities decrease. Focus on increasing carbohydrate consumption in preworkout snacks. You may need higher carbohydrate intake if you are doing a carbohydrate load before a race.	Fat oxidation (breakdown) decreases, which does not warrant any dietary changes.	For all parts of the cycle, focus on calcium, vitamin D, and iron consumption.
Luteal (days 15-28): Estrogen and progesterone rise and then drop just before menstruation.	Energy needs increase by 2.5-11.5%, which could lead to increases of 50-300 or more cal/day.	Protein oxidation (breakdown) increases, leading to possible increased muscle protein breakdown. Focus on increasing protein intake, especially after workouts.	Carbohydrate oxidation rates decrease, which does not warrant any dietary changes.	Fat oxidation (breakdown) increases. Focus on increasing daily fat consumption.	

Pregnancy and Postpartum

One of the biggest mistakes pregnant female endurance athletes make is forgetting to fuel not only themselves but also the baby growing inside them within the context of endurance activities. There is not enough research on pregnant endurance athletes to discuss the specifics of exercise, but many of the macronutrient recommendations for nonpregnant endurance athletes also apply to pregnant athletes. Keep in mind that because you are exercising *and* growing a human, more overall energy intake is required. This can be particularly challenging for women who experience nausea, constipation, and other side effects during pregnancy.

Here are a few things to keep in mind as you embark on your own fitness and nutrition journey as a pregnant athlete:

1. Be sure that the level of training you are doing has been cleared by your health care provider.

2. This applies to all female athletes: never perform a training session while fasted. When you are pregnant, your blood sugar may fluctuate often. Taking in some carbohydrate before exercise is important to prevent hypoglycemic events.

3. Make sure you eat enough for yourself, the baby, and the amount of exercise you're doing. Pregnancy is not the time to skimp on calories; doing so could be harmful to the developing baby.

   a. *First trimester:* You don't need to eat any additional calories besides your base calorie needs plus exercise needs.

   b. *Second trimester:* You need an additional 340 calories besides your base calorie needs plus exercise needs.

   c. *Third trimester:* You need an additional 450 calories besides your base calorie needs plus exercise needs (Academy of Nutrition and Dietetics 2019).

4. Micronutrient requirements increase during pregnancy. Take a prenatal vitamin throughout your pregnancy. Pregnant athletes should pay particular attention to iron, calcium, vitamin D, and all B vitamin levels.

5. It can be difficult to get in enough nutrition as a pregnant athlete when your appetite is lacking. The following tips can help you navigate nausea:

   a. *Test smaller portions:* Eat smaller, more frequent meals so you don't force or overload your system.

b. *Try candy:* Suck on ginger or citrus candies to reduce nausea.

c. *Make elevated smoothies or soups:* Mix higher-calorie options, such as avocado, nuts, seeds, and oils, into your favorite smoothie or soup to increase its nutrient density. Sip or eat slowly to get it all in.

d. *Avoid food triggers:* Pregnancy can cause changes in taste preferences. Don't force yourself to eat any particular foods, and avoid smells that may trigger nausea.

Nutrient Needs While Breastfeeding

Breastfeeding demands huge amounts of energy from a female endurance athlete. An additional 650 calories per day besides your normal caloric requirements (basic nutrition plus exercise) is required. If you don't eat enough during this time, it could leave you with high levels of fatigue and increased risk of stress fractures.

Hydration requirements for breastfeeding athletes start at a baseline of 16 cups (128 ounces or 3.8 liters) per day, plus an additional 16 to 20 ounces (480 to 600 milliliters) of fluid for every hour of exercise. This higher fluid intake is important to support milk production. Luckily, this can include fluid sources besides water, such as dairy and nondairy milk, juice, carbonated water, and smoothies (Academy of Nutrition and Dietetics 2022).

Because of the increased energy demands while breastfeeding, certain micronutrients, particularly calcium and vitamins A, C, and D, must be increased either in the diet or through supplementation so that you don't end up with a deficiency (Horvitz West, Hark, and Deen 2014).

While there is no one known food that can help boost milk production, there are certain nutrition strategies that may help support healthy milk production.

1. Focus on adequate energy intake to support you and the amount of breastfeeding you are doing. Remember that your energy needs are already increased as an endurance athlete and that breastfeeding is an added energy expenditure on top of this.

2. Focus on high-nutrient snacks before and after workouts.

3. Stay hydrated, ensuring that you consume 128 ounces (3.8 liters) plus any fluid lost in sweat when you exercise.

Perimenopausal, Menopausal, and Postmenopausal Nutrition

Going through the transitory stages of perimenopause, menopause, and postmenopause is a normal, yet often frustrating, part of life for female endurance athletes. Unfortunately, there has not been a significant amount of research on female endurance athletes throughout the menopause transition, even though they experience major hormonal and performance changes. During this transition, focus on foundational sports nutrition strategies as well as some of the things we do know about the aging female athlete.

As you enter and go through menopause, your hormones change, and you may observe physical changes—this is normal. Particularly, estrogen and progesterone levels drop and may cause body composition changes, including loss of muscle mass and accumulation of fat stores around the midsection. These changes can be especially concerning for female athletes who were used to their bodies performing and looking a certain way. Other issues you may experience during menopause include sleep disruptions, hunger and fullness dysregulation, and a slowed metabolism.

Even though you might experience some or all of these changes, extreme calorie restriction and underfueling is not the safest or most effective answer. While it's tempting to reduce intake, such restrictions can be detrimental to performance and health. Extremely restrictive diets can lead to an increase in cortisol, the stress hormone (Tomiyama et al. 2010). Cortisol spikes in response to stress throughout the day are normal, but if cortisol levels stay elevated for longer periods, this can cause an increased appetite and subsequent episodes of binge eating or excessive energy intake.

Rather than cutting your intake drastically, focus on these actions that can have a positive effect on your physical, mental, and emotional health.

- *Get adequate protein:* The decrease in estrogen can cause decreased muscle mass and bone mineral density. That's why it is important for women in perimenopause and after to ensure they are meeting their protein requirements of 1.6 to 2.2 grams per kilogram of body weight per day. Protein is known to help prevent age-related muscle mass loss and osteoporosis (Bonjour 2011). Pay particular attention to consuming high-quality BCAAs found in dairy, eggs, meat, and soy products. Consuming protein as soon as possible after exercise can positively influence protein balance and aid in recovery to stop muscle protein breakdown.

- *Increase whole-food carbohydrate sources:* As estrogen decreases, insulin resistance can increase (Yan et al. 2019). Insulin supports blood sugar regulation and helps cells absorb and use carbohydrates for energy production. When insulin resistance occurs, cells don't respond as efficiently to insulin, affecting the body's ability to absorb and use carbohydrates. In this case, it can be helpful to focus on simple carbohydrates such as maple syrup, honey, white bread, rice, and gels one to two hours before and after exercise while including complex carbohydrates such as whole grains, beans, and potatoes as part of your regular nutrient intake.

• *Establish a sleep routine:* Both estrogen and progesterone affect the quality of your sleep. If you struggle in this area, it is important to figure out strategies to improve sleep quality. Create an effective bedtime

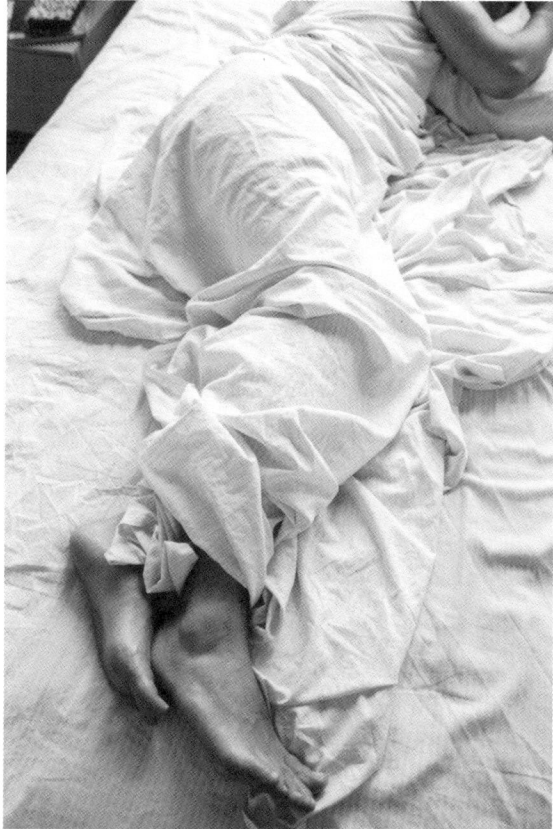

PhotoDisc

A bedtime routine can have a positive effect on your quality of sleep.

routine to wind down at night, keeping your room cool and comfortable, especially if you experience hot flashes. Rather than taking melatonin (long-term use can reduce the body's ability to make melatonin), consider drinking tart cherry juice or a cup of herbal chamomile tea before bed.

• *Hydrate:* With age, thirst cues can decrease, making it challenging to meet hydration needs. It is important to know your fluid loss rate so that you can establish intake patterns that will help you get enough fluid. You may need to use alarms or a schedule to stay hydrated.

• *Pay attention to micronutrients:* Micronutrients of concern during this phase of life include calcium and vitamin D. The decrease in estrogen presents a risk of decreased bone mineral density and osteoporosis. It is recommended that postmenopausal women take in 1,200 milligrams of calcium per day and at least 800 IU of vitamin D per day (Rosen 2023).

Takeaways

- Female endurance athletes have traditionally been given standard nutrition recommendations in line with those of their male counterparts, but we know that women have different physiology throughout their life cycles.

- Nutrition research involving more female athletes continues to evolve, but it is difficult to make conclusions based on a limited number of studies.

- What we do know is summarized in this chapter, but keep in mind that it is always recommended to focus on the basics of endurance sports nutrition first before adjusting the diet with more detailed approaches.

- A recent increase in female athlete study participants will allow for a future that looks at more personalization and periodization throughout the female lifespan.

5

PLANT-BASED ATHLETE FUELING

Running on plants has been a way of life for elite runner and running coach Sage Canaday, who has been a vegetarian since birth. And although he has had a lot of success fueling this way, he emphasizes that being a fully plant-based endurance athlete does require a certain level of dedication and planning to ensure that he gets enough nutrition overall. Ideally, he would like to eat a whole-food, plant-based diet most of the time, but he sometimes finds himself reaching for processed foods that are higher in refined sugars and oil just to get in the calories he needs. He admits that there can be significant challenges as a plant-based athlete if you're not careful and intentional about your fueling choices.

Many endurance athletes were not raised on a plant-based diet but made the switch for ethical reasons or from a desire for better health, recovery, and performance. A 2019 systematic review showed that a short-term (less than 24 months) plant-based diet had positive effects on metabolism, weight, and systemic inflammation, but most of the participants were not athletes (Medawar et al. 2019). Benefits of a plant-based diet may include the following:

- *Improved cardiorespiratory health:* Because a well-planned plant-based diet is high in antioxidants and fiber, this way of eating can offer protective benefits to arterial health, including keeping plaque at bay and allowing for better blood and oxygen flow to the heart and working muscles.

- *Reduced inflammation and enhanced recovery:* Because plants are rich in phytochemicals and have a high amount of antioxidants that scavenge for free radicals, a plant-based diet can help ward off chronic inflammation, which can hinder recovery time, increase injury risk, and increase long-term health risks.

- *More efficient glycogen storage:* Because plant-based foods are typically higher in carbohydrates, they are effective for increasing your glycogen storage after a workout.

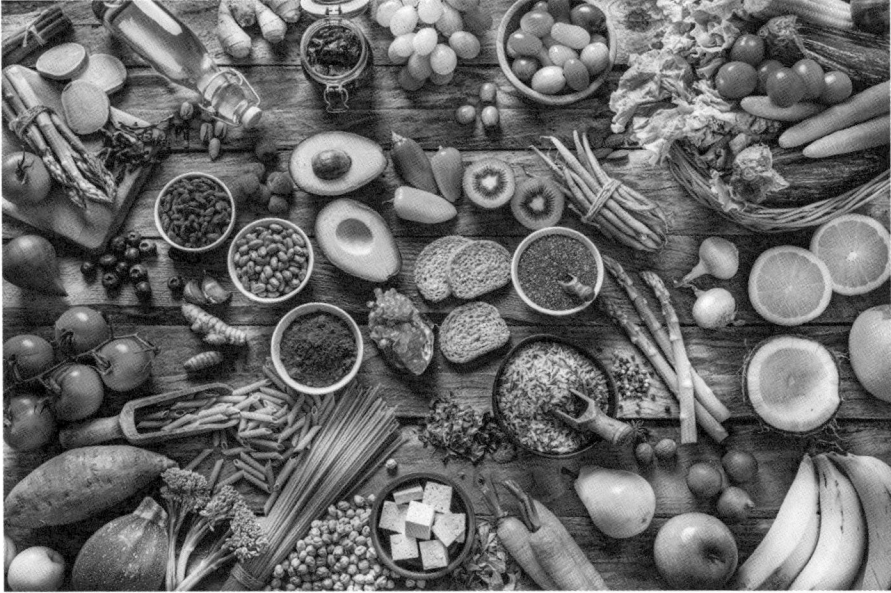

Endurance athletes may switch to a plant-based diet because of a desire for better health, performance, and recovery.

Do a quick search on a plant-based way of eating, and you'll find a whole host of depictions of what this eating style looks like. While there is no standard definition of a plant-based diet, table 5.1 describes the different types of plant-based diets in greater detail. Whatever dietary choices you make, ensure that they fit your lifestyle, beliefs, and performance goals as an endurance athlete.

TABLE 5.1   Types of Plant-Based Diets

Plant-Based Diet	Definition
Vegan	Excludes all animal products such as animal flesh, eggs, dairy, and honey
Vegetarian	Excludes all animal flesh; may or may not allow dairy and eggs
Lacto-vegetarian	Excludes animal flesh and eggs; allows dairy products
Lacto-ovo vegetarian	Excludes animal flesh; allows eggs and dairy products
Ovo vegetarian	Excludes animal flesh and dairy products; allows eggs

Meeting Energy Needs

While well-intentioned, many endurance athletes struggle to figure out the best balance of nutrition on a plant-based diet that will support them in their overall goals. Challenges tend to arise from overall energy deficits as well as macro- and micronutrient deficiencies. Recognizing common deficiencies on a plant-based diet as well as finding strategies to avoid or correct them will help.

Sage Canaday gives one of his biggest pieces of advice to plant-based endurance athletes: Eat bigger portions than you think you might need. Unfortunately, many plant-based endurance athletes who switch to a plant-based diet give up after a few months because they don't get enough overall energy intake. Often, the switch to a plant-based diet entails removing more calorie-dense animal-based foods and replacing them with fruits and vegetables. While fruits and vegetables are rich in micronutrients, they are not dense in calories.

The dangers of underfueling as a plant-based endurance athlete can negate the benefits of gaining training adaptations and increase the risk of fatigue, injury, and illness. Fortunately, including more calorie-dense plant-based foods can help make up for any energy lapses in a plant-based diet, but it may require more intentionality.

How to Boost Energy Intake From Plant-Based Foods

1. *Eat regularly:* Have three meals and three snacks per day with no long gaps between. Aim to eat every two to three hours.
2. *Try a vegan smoothie boost:* Add nut butter and plant-based protein powder to your smoothie to increase the nutrient value.
3. *Consume less fiber:* Switch out high-fiber options for low-fiber choices, such as tofu rather than edamame or white rice instead of brown rice.
4. *Puree your food:* Smoothies and soups are your friend. Liquid nutrition options are always a little easier to get down, especially when you are trying to get a lot in.
5. *Add toppings:* If you're looking for some quick, high-energy additions to incorporate into your plant-based routine, the following food tips can make it easier:

   - Cook with an extra drizzle of oil or vegan butter.
   - Top sandwiches, burgers, wraps, and tacos with avocado, guacamole, or vegan cheese.
   - Put maple syrup or agave on vegan yogurt, pudding, pancakes, waffles, and smoothies.
   - Eat white rice, white pasta, white bread, or rice noodles instead of their high-fiber counterparts.
   - Try dried fruit or juice instead of large portions of fresh fruit.
   - Use high-energy condiments like vegan mayo, vegan ranch dressing, or cranberry sauce.

- Sauté or roast low-fiber veggies instead of high-fiber, fresh veggies.
- Try mock meats such as those made by Tofurky, Beyond Meat, Gardein, or Morningstar Farms.
- Eat fun foods like chips, cookies, cupcakes, muffins, and vegan chocolate.
- Add nut or seed butter to cereal, oats, smoothies, and crackers.

Frequent energy-dense snacks can fill in any gaps that a plant-based endurance athlete might have. All of the following energy-dense snacks contain at least 200 calories and at least two macronutrients:

High-Energy Plant-Based Snacks (each over 200 calories)

- Betty Crocker cupcakes (made with vegan egg replacer) and frosting
- Soy or oat milk with Oreos or Vienna Fingers
- Vegan ice cream (such as Ben & Jerry's vegan flavors)
- Tofurky slices inside a pita with sliced veggies and vegan mayo
- Toasted English muffin with red sauce and vegan mozzarella cheese
- Fruit smoothie with nut butter and vegan protein powder
- Chia pudding made with plant-based milk
- Select Kashi, Nature's Path, or Van's toaster waffles with nut butter and syrup

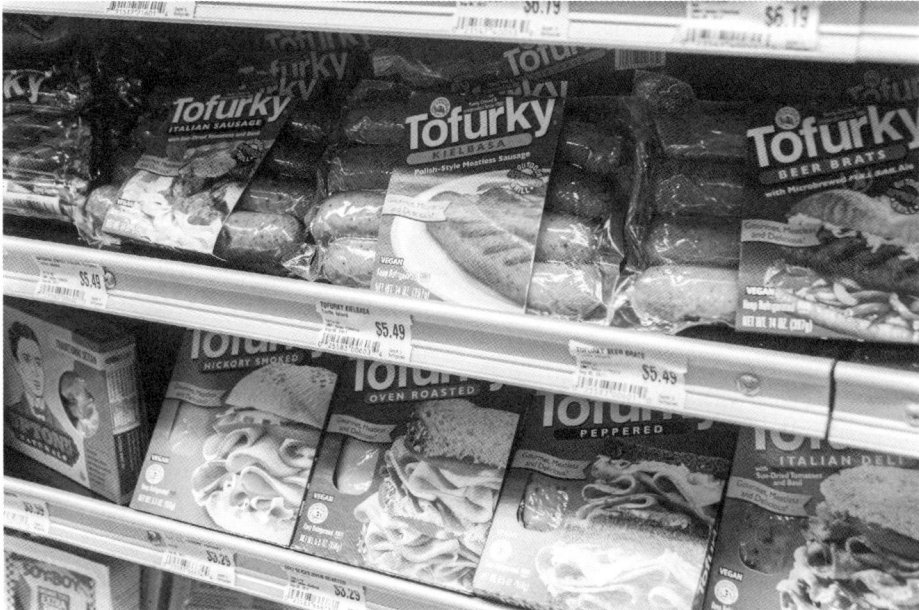

Mock meats, like Tofurky, can be a quick, high-energy addition to your meal planning.

- GoGo Squeez pudding pouch and a handful of crackers
- Can of vegan soup (such as Amy's Kitchen or Gardein) with crackers
- Bagel or English muffin with vegan cream cheese and jam
- Vegan cereal with soy or oat milk and a scoop of nut butter
- Granola bar and nut butter
- Fruit and nut bar or CLIF Bar
- Large apple or banana and nut butter
- Trail mix
- Nut butter and jam sandwich
- Pretzels and hummus
- Tortilla chips and guacamole
- Vegan yogurt with granola or dry cereal
- Vegan cheese or olives with crackers
- Vegan jerky and a large piece of fruit
- Glass of soy milk with vegan chocolate, strawberry, or coffee syrup

Macronutrient Considerations

The reality is that plant-based endurance athletes must be intentional when planning meals and snacks. Macronutrient intake for plant-based endurance athletes tends to prioritize carbohydrate and limit protein. Ideal endurance-specific macronutrient intake may need to be adjusted for a plant-based style of eating due to the sheer volume of food required and limited food options.

Protein

While many plant-based foods do contain some level of protein, the amount of protein is quite variable, and the amino acid profile can be subpar compared to animal protein. Lysine, threonine, cysteine, trypto-phan, methionine, and leucine are the most common amino acids that some plant-based foods are low in. Of particular concern is the BCAA leucine, which plays a key role in maximum muscle protein synthesis rates. Tofu, tempeh, edamame, and soy milk all contain excellent amounts of leucine. While it was previously thought that plant-based athletes needed to consume complementary proteins in the same meal, this has been disproven. Plant-based endurance athletes can meet protein and amino acid needs and support muscle protein synthesis rates by spreading out intake throughout the day and varying protein sources (Shaw et al. 2022).

PRO TIP

Use caution with plant-based protein sources because many of them can be high in fiber. A daily plant-based protein shake may help plant-based endurance athletes meet protein needs, but this should not be overdone.

While reaching protein needs often requires a higher volume of plant-based sources, there are quite a few protein-packed plants. The following are the highest protein-containing plant-based foods.

Top Plant-Based Protein Sources

1. *Seitan:* 3.5 oz (105 g) = 25 g protein
2. *Edamame:* 1 cup (180 g) = 18.4 g protein
3. *Lentils:* 1 cup (200 g), cooked = 18 g protein
4. *Chickpeas:* 1 cup (230 g) = 14.5 g protein
5. *Black beans:* 1 cup (180 g) = 14.2 g protein
6. *Tofu:* 1 cup (230 g) = 12.7 g protein
7. *Hemp seeds:* 3 tbsp = 9 g protein
8. *Quinoa:* 1 cup (185 g), cooked = 8.1 g protein
9. *Peanut butter:* 2 tbsp = 7.2 g protein
10. *Chia seeds:* 1 oz (30 g) = 4.7 g protein

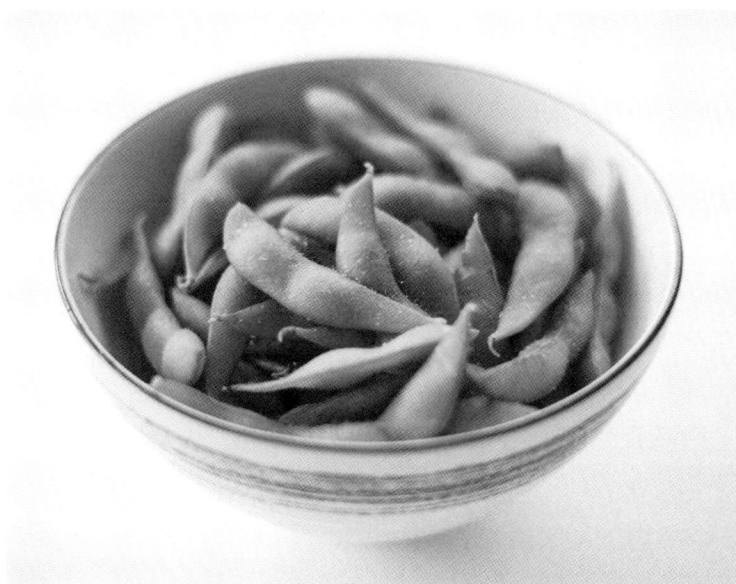

skaman306/Moment RF/Getty Images

Edamame can be a protein-packed source in a plant-based diet.

Protein can be challenging to get, but with a little planning, you can make it happen without too much time or effort. To visualize what a menu might look like, see the following sample meal plans.

Sample Menu for Meeting Protein Needs as a Plant-Based Endurance Athlete Weighing 150 Pounds (68 Kilograms)

Light Day of Training (up to an Hour of Easy Training)

Breakfast: 1 cup (230 g) of oatmeal (cooked), 2 tbsp peanut butter, 8 oz (240 mL) soy milk, blueberries

Snack: 12 oz (360 mL) fruit smoothie made with almond milk and 1 scoop of protein powder

Lunch: Arugula salad with 4 oz (120 g) baked tofu, 1 oz (30 g) pumpkin seeds, 1/2 cup (100 g) quinoa (cooked), and 1/2 cup (115 g) chickpeas

Snack: 2 tbsp hummus with pita and veggies

Dinner: 4 oz (120 g) peanut-baked tempeh with veggies and 1 cup (230 g) cooked rice

Snack: 1 cup (240 mL) soy milk, 1/4 cup (30 g) granola, fruit

Total Protein: about 110 g

Heavy Day of Training (Two to Three Hours of Easy Training)

Breakfast: 2 eggs, 2 pieces of toast topped with 2.5 tbsp peanut butter, banana

Snack: 1 cup (230 g) Greek yogurt with 1/4 cup (30 g) granola and fruit

Lunch: 4 oz (120 g) tempeh and avocado wrap, apple, 8 oz (240 mL) chocolate milk

Snack: 1/2 cup (75 g) shelled edamame, 1 oz (30 g) almonds

Dinner: 1.5 cups (255 g) chickpea pasta (cooked) topped with textured vegetable protein (TVP) tomato "meat" sauce, side salad

Snack: 12 oz (360 mL) fruit smoothie with 1 scoop plant-based protein powder

Total Protein: about 136 g

If you are looking for a quick, high-protein plant-based lunch option, this tofu bowl recipe found here can provide everything you need to fuel a big day.

What About Plant-Based Meats?

With regular meat, you know exactly what nutrition you are getting. Plant-based meat alternatives include products such as burgers, bacon, and crumbles that are formulated to taste like their meat counterparts but are made of soy, vegetable protein, peas, vital wheat gluten, or beans. Many athletes assume these products are healthier because they are plant-based. Whether this is true is up for debate because plant-based meat products contain added fat, sodium, sugar, fillers, and flavorings to get them to taste similar to meat. In fact, a 2021 study published by Tso and Forde in *Nutrients* showed that plant-based diets using plant-based meat alternatives fell short of daily requirements for magnesium, calcium, potassium, zinc, and vitamin B_{12}. The takeaway is that plant-based meat alternatives can be a convenient protein source, but it is important to consider a variety of plant-based protein options to meet protein needs.

Tofu and Rice Bowl With Peanut Sauce

High in protein and carbohydrate, with a little spicy kick, this bowl offers an easy and delicious way to get more plant-based nutrition to meet your unique needs. Servings: 2

Ingredients

- 2/3 cup (130 g) dry basmati rice (rinsed and dried)
- 12 oz (345 g) tofu (extra firm and cubed)
- 1 tbsp oil (divided)
- 1 tbsp soy sauce or tamari (divided)
- Salt and pepper (to taste)
- 1-1/2 tsp arrowroot powder
- 2 cups (320 g) edamame pods (frozen)
- 2 tbsp rice vinegar
- 1/4 tsp chili flakes or chili crunch
- 1/4 cup (60 mL) peanut sauce
- Chopped green onions (for topping)

Directions

1. Preheat oven to 400 °F (200 °C) and line a baking sheet with parchment paper.
2. Cook the rice.
3. Add the tofu cubes to a bowl and gently toss with half the oil and half the soy sauce or tamari. Season with salt and pepper. Add the

arrowroot powder and gently toss until the tofu cubes are well coated. Arrange on the baking sheet. Bake for 15 minutes.

4. Toss the edamame with the remaining oil and soy sauce or tamari and season with salt and pepper. Move the tofu to one side of the baking sheet and add the edamame. Place back in the oven and bake for 12 to 14 minutes or until cooked through and the tofu is crispy.

5. In a small bowl, mix the rice vinegar and chili flakes.

6. Divide the rice, tofu, and edamame into bowls. Top with chopped green onions and drizzle with chili flakes and peanut sauce. Yum!

Carbohydrate and Fiber

Plant-based athletes typically have no problems meeting carbohydrate requirements because protein-rich plant sources are often also high in carbohydrates. On a calorie basis, a plant-based athlete's carbohydrate needs are no different than any other endurance athlete's needs. However, problems arise when they consume too much fiber throughout the day. Fiber is technically a carbohydrate, but our bodies can't digest it and use it as energy. The RDA for fiber is 38 g for men and 25 g for women. While everyone's gastrointestinal tract is different, for some endurance athletes, too much fiber can cause early fullness, bloating, unwanted bathroom breaks, and gastrointestinal distress during workouts. These are not welcome symptoms for athletes who have high energy demands. In some extreme cases, too much fiber is thought to block absorption of certain micronutrients. Phytates and tannins found in plant-based foods can create complexes and chelate, or combine with, minerals and block absorption of those minerals. Beans, grains, and nuts all have higher tannin or phytate content, so consuming too much of these foods can be problematic.

If you want to reach your fiber goal without causing gastrointestinal distress, aim to eat it two to three hours before or after a workout. If you struggle with symptoms of excessive fiber consumption, it may be advantageous to blend or cook fruits, vegetables, and beans to help the digestive process. You can also choose low-fiber simple carbohydrate options for grains, such as white rice instead of brown rice or white pasta instead of whole-wheat pasta.

Additional Tips

1. Avoid high-fiber foods two to three hours before a workout. Remember that everyone's gut is different, so you may need to adjust depending on how your body reacts to high-fiber foods.

2. Avoid high-fiber foods during workouts and races. Note that anything with three or more grams of carbohydrate per serving is considered high fiber.

3. Incorporate low-fiber protein options into your diet rather than relying solely on beans or legumes. For example, you can choose seitan, tofu, soy milk, or mock meats.

Fat

Fatty acid intake in a plant-based diet tends to be lower than in animal-based diets. This is typically because animal products are naturally higher in fat content. Because fats are important energy-dense sources of nutrition for endurance athletes, having a low-fat diet can leave plant-based athletes grasping for energy.

In particular, plant-based diets can have lower intakes of inflammation-balancing omega-3 fatty acids. Emphasize consuming plant-based sources of omega-3s, including chia seeds, flax seeds, and walnuts.

Tips for Transitioning to a Plant-Forward Diet

Slowly transitioning to a plant-forward diet can be a more effective way to make changes than completely overhauling your diet. Depending on your health and performance goals, a plant-forward diet could allow for flexibility, especially during travel or times of high stress. Here are some ways to get started and create an eating pattern that works for you:

1. *Consider having meatless days:* Starting with one or two meatless days each week can help ease you into the plant-based lifestyle without feeling too overwhelmed. This can allow you to explore balanced and satisfying plant-based meals.

2. *Eat animal products on heavy training days only:* Consuming animal products on heavier training days (over two hours) can help you meet higher nutrition requirements (such as with protein) while eating few or no animal products on lighter training days.

3. *Reduce daily animal product consumption by a certain percentage:* Maybe you currently eat animal products at every meal throughout the day. Try decreasing your daily percentage by having meals without any animal products (e.g., going from 100 percent to 50 percent) as a helpful way to start reducing animal product consumption.

4. *Try new plant-based foods each week:* Set a goal to test out a few new plant-based options every week to explore what is out there and what might be your new favorites. For instance, if you have never tried bulgur or amaranth, set a goal to try them twice throughout the week.

5. *Swap your favorite foods for plant-based foods:* Each week, try out plant-based versions of your favorite animal-based staples to see if you can replace them. For instance, try different plant-based milks to see if there is one you like.

Micronutrient Considerations

Plant-based foods are often high in most B vitamins, magnesium, vitamin A, vitamin C, vitamin E, vitamin K, and minerals such as potassium and phosphorus. However, a plant-based diet tends to be lower in vitamin B_{12}, iron, calcium, zinc, and copper.

Vitamin B_{12}

Vitamin B_{12}, or cyanocobalamin, is an essential vitamin that assists in the production of DNA, red blood cells, and the protective sheath around nerve fibers. Cobalamin, the precursor to active B_{12}, is only found in animal products, which puts plant-based athletes at a much higher risk of developing a deficiency. A B_{12} deficiency can lead to a condition called *megaloblastic anemia* in which red blood cells are prevented from dividing, causing the cells to become too large. If the deficiency continues for a long time, athletes become at risk for nerve damage, tingling, numbness, mental confusion, and even paralysis.

It can be difficult to get enough active B_{12} on a plant-based diet. Foods fortified with B_{12} or nutritional yeast grown or cultured in a B_{12} medium are the only reliable sources. Check the labels of your favorite plant-based foods to see if they contain B_{12} fortification. Cereals, tempeh, and plant milks are the most common places it is found.

> **PRO TIP**
>
> Be wary of claims that suggest plant-based foods such as shiitake mushrooms, sea vegetables, and tempeh contain B_{12}. These foods contain an inactive form of B_{12} that the body cannot use. You may want to consider B_{12} supplementation as a plant-based athlete to avoid risking deficiency.

Iron

Endurance athletes lose iron in many ways—through sweat, urine, the gastrointestinal tract, and menstruation—making their iron requirements higher than that of the average person. A plant-based endurance athlete's iron requirements are even higher, and they are advised to take in nearly two times the recommended daily value (National Institutes of Health 2023). This is because plant-based iron is a form called *nonheme iron*. Nonheme iron accounts for more than 80 percent of standard daily iron intake, but it has a poor absorption rate of only 1 to 12 percent (Chouraqui 2022). Comparatively speaking, heme iron, which comes from animal-based sources, is absorbed at a rate of 15 to 35 percent, depending on a person's iron stores (Monsen 1988).

To get enough plant-based iron in the diet, it is important to understand which plant-based foods contain the most iron and how much of those foods you need to eat to get enough iron to support your plant-based athlete lifestyle. The following plant-based foods contain the highest iron amounts.

Top Plant-Based Foods Containing Iron

1. *Lentils:* 1 cup (200 g), cooked = 6.6 mg iron
2. *Tofu:* 1/2 cup (115 g) = 6.6 mg iron
3. *Spinach:* 1 cup (180 g), cooked = 6.43 mg iron
4. *Kidney beans:* 1 cup (225 g), cooked = 5.2-6.6 mg iron
5. *Amaranth:* 1 cup (250 g), cooked = 5.1 mg iron
6. *Dark chocolate:* 1 oz (30 g) = 3.4 mg iron
7. *White mushrooms:* 1 cup (175 g), cooked = 2.7 mg iron
8. *Hemp seeds:* 3 tbsp = 2.3 mg iron
9. *White potato:* 1 medium = 2 mg iron
10. *Dried apricots:* 1/2 cup (85 g) = 2 mg iron

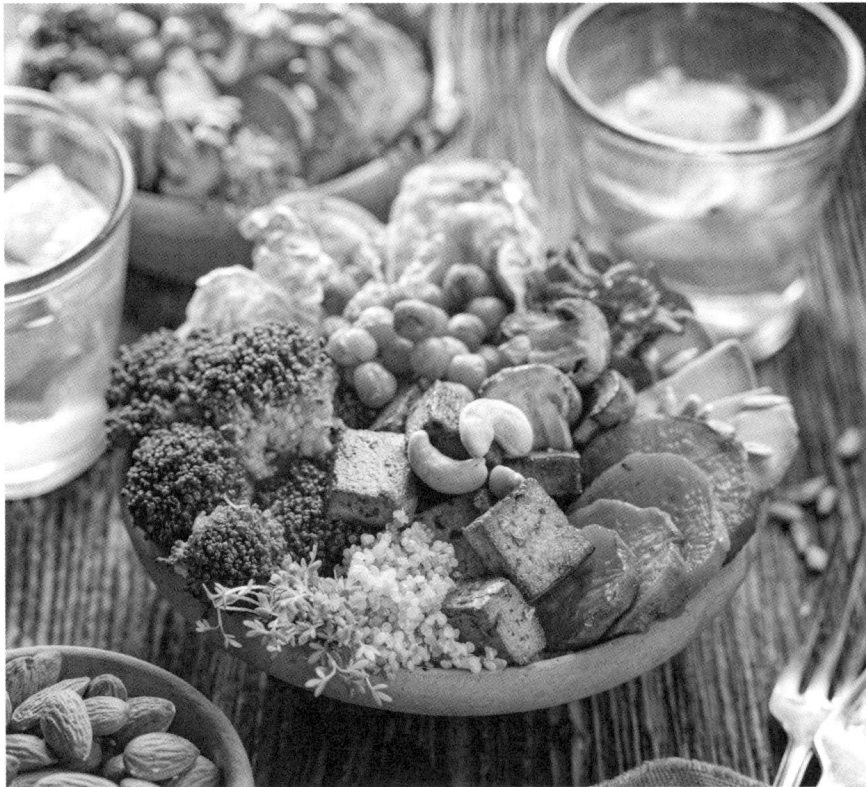

zi3000/iStockphoto/Getty Images

Tofu provides a high amount of iron for a plant-based diet.

PRO TIP

Try to find simple solutions to increase overall iron intake from a few foods instead of many different foods. For instance, including a high-iron smoothie or a cup of iron-fortified cereal every day might be a more convenient way for you to meet your iron needs than trying to include a wide range of iron-rich foods.

If you're looking for a convenient way to get a high amount of plant-based iron in one meal, try the smoothie bowl recipe listed here.

Mixed Berry Beet Smoothie Bowl

This plant-based smoothie is a good source of iron.
Servings: 1

Ingredients

- 1 cup (150 g) mixed frozen berries
- 1/2 fresh beet (chopped, frozen)
- 2 tbsp pitted dates
- 1/2 cup (120 mL) soy milk
- 1/4 cup (40 g) chia seeds
- 1 tbsp unsweetened coconut flakes
- 1 tbsp 80% cacao chocolate chips
- 1 tbsp chopped pecans

Directions

1. Combine soy milk, dates, frozen berries, and beet into a blender and blend until smooth.
2. Pour smoothie mixture into a bowl and top with coconut flakes, chia seeds, chocolate chips, and pecans.
3. Top with fresh berries if desired.

Calcium

While the Academy of Nutrition and Dietetics considers calcium a nutrient of concern for plant-based athletes, with a little bit of planning, you can find plenty of plant-based calcium sources that the body can use. Choosing plant-based calcium sources that are lower in oxalates can help support absorption. Oxalates, or oxalic acid, can bind to minerals in the digestive system and block absorption of those minerals. For example, spinach is high in calcium and oxalate, which prevents a large amount of the calcium from being absorbed into the body. Bok choy and kale contain high levels of calcium but low levels of oxalate, which make them better overall plant-based sources of calcium. The following plant-based foods are high in calcium but low in oxalates to help you get the most out of what you are consuming.

Top Plant-Based Foods Containing Calcium

1. *Fortified orange juice:* 1 cup (240 mL) = 350 mg calcium
2. *Oat milk:* 1 cup (240 mL) = 350 mg calcium
3. *Blackstrap molasses:* 1 tbsp = 200 mg calcium
4. *Bok choy:* 1 cup (70 g), raw = 158 mg calcium
5. *Kale:* 1 cup (25 g), raw = 90 mg calcium
6. *Broccoli:* 1 cup (90 g) = 70 mg calcium

Zinc

Zinc plays a key role in immune function, healing, and cellular enzyme reactions. As with iron, plant-based sources of zinc contain phytates, or phytic acid, which can block the absorption of zinc. Soaking and sprouting beans, grains, nuts, and seeds can help reduce the negative impact of phytates on absorption and increase the bioavailability of zinc (Shaw et al. 2022). Because of reduced bioavailability, the recommended zinc intake for plant-based athletes is 50 percent higher than the standard recommendation: 12 milligrams per day for women and 16.5 milligrams per day for men (Tso and Forde 2021).

The following plant-based foods are highest in zinc content. Please note that they all contain some phytic acid, which is why plant-based athletes are advised to consume higher amounts per day than the standard recommendations.

Top Plant-Based Foods Containing Zinc

1. *Fortified cereal:* 3/4 cup (45 g) = about 19 mg zinc (170% Daily Value [DV])
2. *Oats:* 1 cup dry (80 g) = 6.2 mg zinc (56% DV)
3. *Tofu:* 1 cup (230 g) = 4 mg zinc (36% DV)
4. *Wheat germ:* 1 oz (30 g) = 4.7 mg zinc (43% DV)
5. *Hemp seeds:* 1 oz (30 g) = 2.8 mg zinc (26% DV)

Copper

Copper is important for iron metabolism, hemoglobin production, and energy metabolism. While copper is prevalent in a variety of plant-based foods, some mineral-to-mineral interactions with zinc and phytate activity can inhibit its absorption. Like with zinc-rich foods, soaking and sprouting copper-rich foods before eating them can help increase the bioavailability of copper.

Because of copper's key role in iron absorption and the transfer of iron from the intestinal mucosa to the blood plasma, it is important to make sure you are getting in enough copper daily. The RDA for copper is 900 micrograms, but while studies have demonstrated that exercise increases the need for this micronutrient, it is unclear how much of an increase is sufficient to maintain blood plasma and intracellular copper status (Rakhra et al. 2021). The following are some of the highest plant-based sources of copper.

Top Plant-Based Foods Containing Copper

1. *Tofu:* 1 cup (230 g) = 1 mg copper (106% DV)
2. *Sweet potatoes:* 1 cup (230 g) = 0.7 mg copper (79% DV)
3. *Cashews:* 1 oz (30 g) = 0.6 mg copper (70% DV)
4. *Chickpeas:* 1 cup (230 g), cooked = 0.6 mg copper (64% DV)
5. *Dark chocolate:* 1 oz (30 g) = 0.5 mg copper (56% DV)

Takeaways

- Taking part in a plant-based style of eating has different meanings for different endurance athletes.
- Plant-based eating requires more planning, effort, and food volume to ensure that you're meeting macronutrient and micronutrient needs.
- Before making the switch to a plant-based diet, weigh the benefits and risks, and consider your lifestyle.
- Sometimes easing into a plant-forward diet first can help you make changes and adjust without it feeling too extreme.
- It can also be helpful to check on yourself regularly to ensure you are getting enough macronutrients and micronutrients to support your level of training.
- Consider annual blood panels for micronutrients of concern for plant-based endurance athletes (see recommendations above).

SPECIAL DIETARY NEEDS

I was diagnosed with celiac at age 16. At first, it felt incredibly restrictive and completely inaccessible as an athlete—that and the early beginnings of low-carb/paleo, it was the absolute most perfect environment for me to lean myself up into a full-blown eating disorder. The misinformation was confusing for me—as a teenager and as an athlete. Not only did it feel difficult to fuel well for my sport, it was socially disruptive: from needing special snacks or meals to choosing where to stop to eat on a team trip—at some level, my diet became everyone else's problem (or so it felt at 16). Even as an adult, the where-to-eat question revolves around me.

Fueling strategies have improved dramatically in the last 20 years, but not planning or preparing is simply not an option. Long rides supported by gas stations are a no. Even coffee shops and small-town grocery stores can be hit or miss. Eating out has its challenges with cross-contamination and understanding of what celiac means. I've found that traveling for sport with celiac is also an agility course of its own—different languages, different packaging, different processing. It's just not as easy as stopping at Subway for lunch, banking on dinner that isn't salad for dinner. And yes, it does feel sad to skip the pizza in Italy!

Ultimately, it comes down to preparation, ensuring that I travel with the nutrition I need to perform the way I want to perform. I cannot underfuel if I'm overprepared; this has become my complete ethos around training, racing, and traveling with celiac.

—Bernie Nelson, Head Team Comp Coach ASC Training Center, Former U.S. Ski Team Coach and Elite Nordic Skier (interview, 2024)

You likely know (or are) someone who has eliminated a range of foods from their diet to determine if they have food allergies. Many times, these food eliminations lead endurance athletes to include only a small number of "safe" foods in their diet to try and figure out what (if anything) could help them feel better holistically. Studies have shown that 30 to 50 percent of the gastrointestinal issues endurance athletes experience are common in the population (de Oliveira, Burini, and Jeukendrup 2014). Many people claim that eliminating certain foods reduces joint pain, enhances recovery, and cures ailments. While elimination diets can be helpful when conducted under the guidance of a registered dietitian or health care professional, too often they can cause the unnecessary removal of certain foods and food groups that are crucial to endurance training, which can leave endurance athletes at higher risk of underfueling and malnutrition.

Food allergies are a very real thing. However, the prevalence of true food allergies is likely a lot lower than the general public thinks. Food intolerances, however, are quite common and can cause symptoms similar to those brought on by food allergies. That brings us to this question: How can we accurately determine what is a food allergy and what is an intolerance, and how do we then create a fueling strategy that supports overall health and performance?

Food Allergies Versus Food Intolerances

The first distinction we must make is between food allergies and food intolerances. Adverse reactions to food can be classified as allergies or intolerance, and because of this, both terms tend to be used interchangeably, causing confusion for many. The difference between the two is that a true allergy incites an immunoglobulin E (IgE) immune system response stemming from the protein-containing portion of the food, while an intolerance causes a reaction (nonimmune system response) to any component of the food (Crowe 2019). It is important to distinguish what kind of response you are having to particular foods; if you don't, it can lead to the unnecessary removal of entire food groups that you may not have problems with and that are crucial to an endurance-athlete diet.

Food allergies and intolerances most commonly develop in childhood, but about 15 percent of food allergies develop in adulthood. Rates of food intolerance are reportedly as high as 20 to 25% percent of the worldwide population, but it can be hard to distinguish between food allergy and intolerance due to overlapping symptoms (Crowe 2019). The most common symptoms of food allergies and intolerances include diarrhea, constipation, bloating, cramping, nausea, and upset stomach. Those with more serious food allergies may have more severe symptoms like anaphylaxis, hives, and trouble breathing.

True food allergy and sensitivity testing can be a confusing process. There are many over-the-counter options available for purchase, but many of these tests use immunoglobulin G (IgG), immunoglobulin A (IgA), and cytotoxicity; lack standardization; and are not recommended. The gold standard for food allergy testing is IgE blood testing, along with a skin prick test and oral food challenges. These tests should all be done by a trained allergist. The top nine most common food allergies are milk, wheat, soy, eggs, peanuts, corn, tree nuts, fish or shellfish, and sesame—these make up 90 percent of the world's food allergies (U.S. Food and Drug Administration 2023).

To test for food sensitivities, the best way is to use an elimination diet to remove suspected foods one at a time and look for symptom improvement. Athletes must take care during an elimination diet to avoid significant nutrient deficiencies.

Endurance Athletes and Navigating Special Diets

If you have allergies or sensitivities as an endurance athlete, it might be inconvenient, but you can make it through if you plan ahead and take the following factors into consideration:

1. *Race fueling strategy:* If you have special diet considerations, it is very important that you have a fueling plan and do not rely on racecourse nutrition. For instance, if you have celiac disease and cannot tolerate gluten, bring gluten-free sports nutrition products and foods with you instead of relying on the race organizers to accommodate your needs.

2. *Overall energy intake:* Having food allergies and sensitivities can make it difficult to get all the energy intake you need as an endurance athlete, especially if you have more than one food you must avoid. Be sure to evaluate your overall energy intake regularly to ensure that you are not unintentionally underfueling.

3. *Gastrointestinal stress:* Food allergies and intolerances can leave athletes feeling bloated, in pain, or under constant gastrointestinal distress during training sessions. Consuming the offending foods can cause inflammation and an immune response in the body, which can leave athletes struggling. Make sure you are completely removing offending foods so your gastrointestinal tract can stay healthy.

Common Food Intolerances and Special Diets

If an endurance athlete is diagnosed with a food allergy or intolerance, they may need to follow a restrictive diet for a short or extended time in order to feel better. These special diets require more careful planning and monitoring so that overall calorie and micronutrient needs are met to support training demands. There is a wide range of food allergies and sensitivities that may affect endurance athletes. Let's look at some of the most common.

Gluten-Related Intolerances (Celiac or Nonceliac Gluten Sensitivity)

There are three disorders associated with gluten intolerance: true celiac disease, nonceliac gluten sensitivity, and wheat allergy. Gluten itself is a family of proteins found in grains and includes both glutenin and glia-din. In some people, these proteins can cross the gut lining and cause an immune response, inducing inflammatory processes and symptoms such as diarrhea, bloating, anaphylaxis, skin issues, and constipation (Roszkowska et al. 2019).

Diagnosis of celiac disease is first performed using either serology testing, which looks for antibodies in the blood, or genetic testing for human leukocyte antigens (HLA-DQ2 and HLA-DQ8). If either of these tests comes back positive, a more invasive endoscopy or capsule endos-copy will be ordered for final diagnosis.

Nonceliac gluten sensitivity is subject to uncertainty when trying to diagnose because of its similarities to irritable bowel syndrome (IBS) and Crohn's disease. Currently, the best way to diagnose nonceliac gluten sensitivity is to completely remove gluten from the diet for six weeks, monitor symptoms along the way, then reintroduce gluten and monitor symptoms again.

If you determine that gluten is a real issue for you and you need to remove it completely, it is important to have a good understanding of what foods contain gluten, even hidden sources of gluten. See table 6.1 for gluten-containing foods and table 6.2 for non-gluten-containing foods.

TABLE 6.1   Gluten-Containing Foods

Wheat bread	Pretzels	Barley malt	Oats (need to be certified gluten-free, but even those may not be safe for those who also cannot tolerate a protein in oats simi-lar to gluten called *avenin*)
Cereal	Bread	Graham flour	Oat groats
Crackers	Barley	Bran	Bread flour
Croutons	Kamut	High-protein flour	Rye flour
Pasta	Triticale	Bulgur	Couscous
Soba noodles	Durum flour	Wheat flour	Farina
Wheat germ	Farro	White flour	Beer made with barley
Malt syrup or vinegar	Candy	Matzo meal	Deli meat

Meatballs	Flavored coffees	Muffins	Gravies
Salad dressings	Hamburger patties	Sauces	Hot dogs
Soup	Inulin	Frozen meals	Ketchup
Ice cream	Soy sauce	Malted milk	Teriyaki sauce
Breaded foods	Seasoned rice		

TABLE 6.2 Non-Gluten-Containing Foods

Amaranth	Sago	Potato flour	Wine and other spirits (except beer and whiskey)
Quinoa	Tapioca flour	Yam flour	Meats
Buckwheat	Mesquite flour	Beans	Dairy
Brown rice	Arrowroot flour	Nuts	Fruits and vegetables
Rice flour	Millet	Seeds	
Chickpea flour	Teff	Butter and oil	

Issues with gluten can cause damage to intestinal cells, which can lead to deficiencies in certain micronutrients. Specifically, athletes should be aware of minerals (particularly iron and magnesium), and vitamins A, D, E, and K. Deficiencies in these micronutrients may require supplementation if intake cannot be achieved through the diet.

Tree Nut and Peanut Allergies

Tree nuts and peanuts are often grouped together as one allergy category because their allergic reactions can overlap. Tree nuts include cashews, almonds, walnuts, hazelnuts, Brazil nuts, and pine nuts. Peanuts are not true nuts; they are legumes. Tree nut and peanut allergies occur when the body reacts to the proteins in the nuts, leading to symptoms throughout the body, such as rashes, respiratory distress, gastrointestinal stress, and anaphylaxis. Some athletes may react to only one type of nut, while others may react to many.

Depending on the severity of the allergy, tree nut and peanut allergies can be tricky to navigate because many foods and sports nutrition products are made in facilities that process nuts. Take great care to read labels when choosing food and sports nutrition products. For athletes who have a tree nut or peanut allergy, it is helpful to carry an EpiPen in case of accidental exposure.

If you are an endurance athlete who cannot use nuts as a convenient low-volume option to get in extra calories and fats, consider the following seed options instead.

Alternatives for a Nut-Free Diet
- Sunflower seeds and sunflower seed butter
- Chia seeds
- Tahini
- Sesame seeds
- Hemp seeds
- Pumpkin seeds and pumpkin seed butter
- Flax seeds
- Watermelon seeds and watermelon seed butter

Dairy Allergy and Lactose Intolerance

When discussing a dairy allergy, it is important to distinguish between a true allergy to proteins found in cow's milk products and lactose intolerance, which is caused by an insufficient production of lactase. A dairy allergy can lead to systemic immune effects like skin issues, anaphylaxis, and respiratory issues, while lactose intolerance can lead to gastrointestinal symptoms like diarrhea, gas, and bloating.

Navigating a dairy-free diet as an endurance athlete can be a relatively simple process if you understand common dairy-free alternatives and possible deficiencies that can occur when you're not consuming dairy

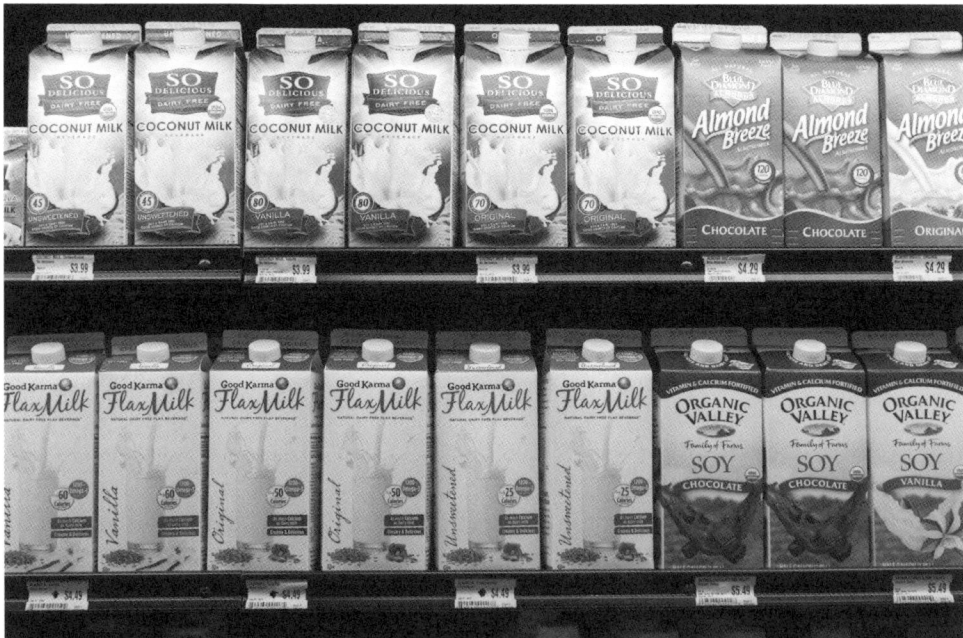

Fortified soy, almond, and oat milk provide dairy-free alternatives to dairy milk.

products. The most common nutrients that come from dairy products are protein, calcium, and vitamin D (see table 6.3). It is important for athletes to find alternative sources of these nutrients so they can meet dietary needs.

TABLE 6.3   Common Nutrients Found in Dairy Products

Dairy-Free Protein Sources	Dairy-Free Calcium Sources	Dairy-Free Vitamin D Sources
Meats	Leafy greens	Fatty fish
Beans	Fortified orange juice	Irradiated mushrooms
Lentils	Fortified soy, almond, and oat milks	Fortified soy, almond, and oat milks
Chickpeas	Tofu	
Tofu	Almonds	
Tempeh	Chia seeds	
Quinoa	Alternative milk yogurts	

A Note on Reading Labels

It is important for endurance athletes with a true dairy allergy to read food labels and look for hidden sources of dairy. Even if a label states that a product is dairy-free, take care to double-check the ingredients list. The same holds true for any food you want to avoid: It may not be obvious that a substance is present in a food, so it's always best to check the label.

Hidden Dairy Terms to Look Out for

Casein and caseinates

Whey

Lactose

Lactalbumin

Milk by-products

Curd

Ghee

Rennet casein

The Low-FODMAP Diet

FODMAPs may be harder for some athletes to digest and absorb in the small intestine. The low-FODMAP diet is designed to manage IBS. While diagnostic criteria differs between IBS and FODMAP intolerance, IBS affects about 11 percent of the global population (Canavan, West, and

Card 2014). FODMAPs include a family of carbohydrates that are poorly absorbed in the small intestine and then fermented in the large intestine, which can lead to uncomfortable gastrointestinal symptoms such as gas, bloating, diarrhea, and constipation. The low-FODMAP diet itself is not a diet in the traditional restrictive sense, but rather a three-part clinical approach developed by Monash University in Australia to help uncover individual FODMAP tolerance. This approach is not meant to cure underlying gastrointestinal disease, but rather relieve symptoms.

What Are FODMAPs?

Let's break down the individual carbohydrates that make up FODMAPs:

1. *Oligosaccharides:* This group includes fructans and galacto-oligosaccharides, found in foods such as wheat, onions, garlic, and legumes.

2. *Disaccharides:* Lactose is the main disaccharide in this group, found in the following foods:
   - Yogurt
   - Cow's milk
   - Sheep's milk
   - Goat's milk
   - Soft cheeses
   - Ice cream
   - Sour cream
   - Kefir
   - Cream cheese

3. *Monosaccharides:* This group is primarily fructose, found in high amounts in honey, certain fruits, and high-fructose corn syrup. High-fructose foods include the following:
   - Apples
   - Pears
   - Mangoes
   - Cherries
   - Figs
   - Pears
   - Watermelon
   - Dried fruit
   - Fruit juices
   - Molasses

- Asparagus
- Peas

4. *Polyols:* Sugar alcohols like sorbitol and mannitol make up the majority of this group and can be found in some fruits, vegetables, and artificial sweeteners. High-polyol foods include the following:
   - Apples
   - Avocados
   - Plums
   - Green bell peppers
   - Peaches
   - Cherries
   - Mushrooms
   - Celery
   - Sweet potatoes
   - Sugar-free gums, candies, and ice creams

If you've determined you have IBS and want to see if a low-FODMAP diet may be helpful for you, here's a suggested implementation strategy. As an endurance athlete, you may want to work closely with a sports dietitian to help you through each step in the process and ensure you are performing it correctly.

1. *Restriction phase (two to six weeks):* All high-FODMAP foods are eliminated from the diet to see if symptoms reduce.

2. *Reintroduction phase (length varies):* High-FODMAP foods are reintroduced methodically, one at a time, to identify which FODMAP foods and amounts are tolerable.

3. *Long-term phase (ongoing):* FODMAP foods that cannot be tolerated are kept out of the diet or are limited to small amounts.

Keep in mind that the low-FODMAP diet is meant to be a temporary elimination diet to figure out which foods may be exacerbating gastro-intestinal symptoms. Long-term strict elimination of all FODMAP foods, such as the restriction phase described above, can lead to malnutrition and micronutrient deficiencies in endurance athletes. There is no ideal length of time for the diet, but it is important to follow a similar timeline to the one that was previously presented.

Implementing the low-FODMAP diet requires knowledge of which foods contain high amounts of FODMAPs. Monash University has a website and app that are helpful tools for identifying high- and low-FODMAP foods. Use table 6.4 to help you decipher between low and high FODMAP foods.

TABLE 6.4   **High- and Low-FODMAP Foods**

Type of food	High-FODMAP foods	Low-FODMAP foods
Fruits	Apples, cherries, nectarines, dried fruits, peaches, plums, and watermelon	Cantaloupe, kiwis, oranges, and pineapples
Vegetables	Asparagus, green peas, onions, garlic, and mushrooms	Eggplant, green beans, bok choy, carrots, lettuce, potatoes, and zucchini
Dairy and dairy alternatives	Cow's milk, yogurt, and soy milk (made from soybeans)	Almond milk, feta cheese, hard cheeses, lactose-free milk, soy milk (made from soy protein)
Breads, cereals, and grains	Wheat-, barley-, and rye-based breads, cereals, and biscuits	Corn flakes, quinoa, oats, and wheat-, barley-, and rye-free breads
Nuts and seeds	Cashews and pistachios	Peanuts, pumpkin seeds, macadamia nuts, and walnuts
Protein sources	Most beans	Eggs; firm tofu; tempeh; and plain meats, poultry, and seafood
Sweeteners	Honey and high-fructose corn syrup	Maple syrup, rice malt syrup, and table sugar

Source: Department of Gastroenterology, Monash University. This table was reproduced with permission from Monash University (monashfodmap.com). Download the Monash University FODMAP Diet App for FODMAP ratings and serving sizes.

A 2019 study published in the *Journal of the International Society of Sports Nutrition* found that even a short-term low-FODMAP diet improved gastrointestinal symptoms in recreational runners (Wiffin et al. 2019). Gastrointestinal symptoms such as pain, bloating, diarrhea, and nausea are common side effects during endurance training and racing that can lead to unwanted stops. High-FODMAP foods can exacerbate these symptoms because they sit in the system and cause excessive gas production and concentration gradient differences, leading to fluid retention in the small intestine. Research on this diet and its use for endurance athletes is in its infancy.

Challenges of the Low-FODMAP Diet for Endurance Athletes

Sticking to a low-FODMAP diet can be particularly challenging for endurance athletes, especially if time to prepare meals and snacks is limited. Prepackaged foods and convenience items often contain high amounts of FODMAPs, so take care to read labels. If not done appropriately, the low-FODMAP diet can make it difficult to get enough overall calories and micronutrients (particularly B vitamins and calcium) to support training and performance in endurance athletes, leading to more harm than good.

Sports nutrition products used during training often contain high-FOD-MAP ingredients such as fructose, which can make it challenging to navigate race fueling plans. Purchasing glucose-only products or making homemade fueling options may be the best strategy to avoid foods that cause problems. See table 6.5 for low-FODMAP grocery staples to add to your diet.

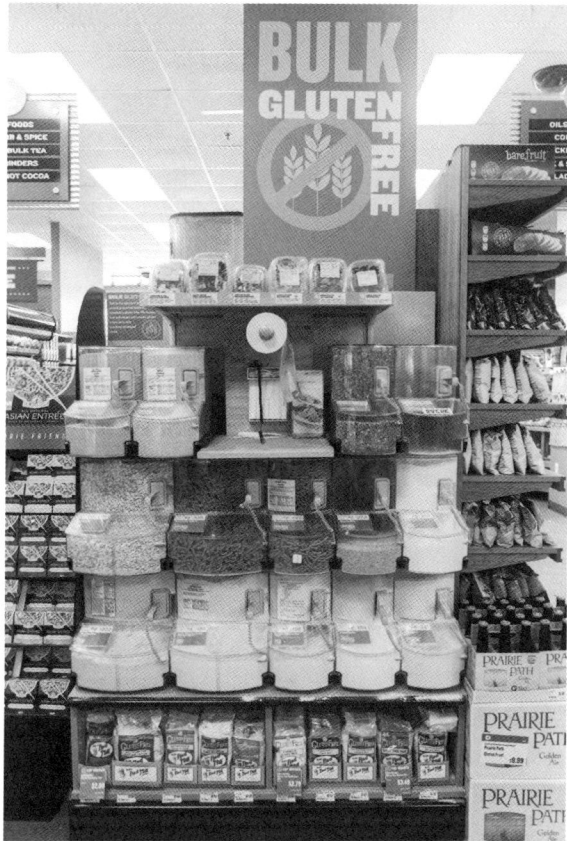

Gluten-free pasta provides endurance athletes with a low-FODMAP alternative to pasta with gluten.

TABLE 6.5   Low-FODMAP Grocery Staples for Athletes

Type of food	Examples of low-FODMAP items
Grains	Rice noodles, gluten-free pasta, spelt sourdough, gluten-free bread, quinoa, oats, and rice
Dairy and dairy alternatives	Lactose-free yogurt, soy milk, almond milk, and firm cheeses
Proteins	Meat, chicken, fish, eggs, firm tofu, canned legumes, seeds, walnuts, and Brazil nuts
Vegetables	Eggplant, green beans, bok choy, broccoli, carrots, cucumbers, lettuce, potatoes, tomatoes, and zucchini
Fruits	Cantaloupe, kiwis, oranges, pineapples, firm bananas, blueberries, and raspberries
Oils and fats	Olive oil, garlic-infused olive oil, and butter
Condiments and sauces	Mustard, peanut butter, soy sauce, tahini, tomato sauce, vinegars, Worcestershire sauce, and miso paste

What follows is a two-day sample menu for the low-FODMAP diet. Because of the high energy needs of endurance athletes, this menu includes frequent meals and snacks.

Sample Low-FODMAP Menu: Day One

Breakfast: Peanut butter chocolate chip overnight oats

Snack 1: Gluten-free crackers with cheese

Lunch: Ground turkey with spinach, acorn squash, and rice

Snack 2: Clementines and macadamia nuts

Dinner: Slow-cooker mustard chicken with rice or gluten-free toast

Snack 3: Pineapple orange smoothie made with lactose-free milk

Sample Low-FODMAP Menu: Day Two

Breakfast: Fried eggs with two slices of gluten-free toast and a side of blueberries

Snack 1: Rice crackers with peanut butter

Lunch: Buffalo quinoa chicken wrap with a side of kiwi (use a gluten-free tortilla and low-FODMAP hot sauce)

Snack 2: Lactose-free yogurt with strawberries

Dinner: Crispy tofu with carrots and rice

Snack 3: Peanut butter chocolate chip GoMacro bar

If you are looking for some tasty low-FODMAP meal and snack ideas that can fuel you up for your training sessions look no further than the recipes listed here.

Peanut Butter Chocolate Chip Overnight Oats

Servings: 1

Ingredients

- 1/2 cup (40 g) dry oats (quick or rolled)
- 1/2 cup (120 mL) unsweetened almond milk
- 1-1/3 tbsp peanut butter
- 2 tsp chia seeds
- 2 tsp maple syrup
- 1 tsp cocoa powder
- 2-2/3 tbsp water

Directions

Combine all ingredients and mix well. Store in refrigerator overnight before consuming.

Pineapple Orange Smoothie

Servings: 1

Ingredients

- 3/4 cup (120 g) frozen pineapple
- Juice from one navel orange
- Zest from one navel orange
- 1/2 cup (120 g) lactose-free yogurt
- 1/4 cup (60 mL) lactose-free milk
- 1/3 cup (45 g) ice

Directions

Combine all ingredients in a blender and blend until smooth.

Takeaways

- True food allergies are seemingly much less common than projected in the media.
- If you have common food-allergy symptoms like gastrointestinal distress, sneezing, coughing, or skin conditions, see an allergist for diagnosis or try a strict, guided elimination diet to identify causes.
- At-home food sensitivity testing is not a reliable way to determine true food allergies and can cause unnecessary fear and anxiety around foods, which can lead to malnutrition in endurance athletes because of their higher nutrient needs.
- Elimination diets are the best way to determine food-sensitivity issues.
- And if you have to remove foods from your diet, be intentional about planning and implementing the changes to ensure you can keep fueling and performing well.

7

PLANNING MEALS AND SNACKS

The first few years into his professional career, Matt Hanson performed well at the beginning of the season but struggled to perform later in the year at the Ironman World Championship. He thought that hunger and fullness were good indicators of whether he was fueling himself well. However, his weight continued to drop throughout every season. It was crucial for Hanson to learn how to fuel himself properly to match his training volume and intensity. Once he created a strategy for maintaining his weight, he was able to excel at the Ironman World Championship.

For many endurance athletes, it's not a lack of knowledge that prevents them from eating to support their goals. With an athlete's career, family, social time, and training, cooking and meal planning might be the last thing on their mind. The idea of planning when and what to eat and prepping it is daunting and often becomes a roadblock rather than an aid. This is where the practicality of this book comes in. You can have all the scientific knowledge in the world, but if you want to execute it properly, you have to put the principles into practice in a way that makes sense for you and your lifestyle. For Hanson, this required him to be more intentional about knowing *what* his body needed and *how* he was going to get it all in.

I like to tell athletes that they need to get away from the idea of having the perfectly balanced performance plate or macronutrient meal all the time, as well as the idea that they have to meal prep for 12 hours on a Sunday to fuel their body well for performance. Overanalyzing the planning and fueling process can lead to failure. The obsession with what to eat often takes precedence over just eating, and many athletes simply don't meet their nutritional needs.

Fueling Tips

Remember, recommendations and numbers are just that. The process of meal planning must be unique to you—and only you—and your situation.

There are many approaches to figuring out what works to meet your fueling demands. The key is to find time-savers, go-tos, and things to help you adapt in the moment if needed.

Before getting started with the planning and shopping process, keep these fueling tips in mind:

1. *Do not skip meals:* Yes, this means eating at regular intervals throughout the day, even when you are busy, stressed, tired, or not hungry. In my experience, the less structure an endurance athlete has around their eating, the more trouble they will have meeting their nutrition needs. If remembering to eat is a challenge, think about setting up windows of time for yourself throughout the day that will help you just get something in. This doesn't mean you have to eat at 8:33 a.m. on the dot every day, but you can set up windows such as the following:

- 5:00 a.m.: Snack 1, before workout
- 7:00 a.m. to 9:00 a.m.: Meal 1
- 12:00 p.m. to 2:00 p.m.: Meal 2
- 2:00 p.m. to 4:00 p.m.: Snack 2
- 5:00 p.m. to 7:00 p.m.: Meal 3
- 9:00 p.m.: Snack 3, before bed

If you know you won't remember to eat something during those times, set alarms on your phone or pop-ups on your computer.

2. *Use snacks as a vehicle for added nutrition:* Are you having trouble meeting nutrition needs with just meals, especially on heavier training days? Think about increasing the number of snacks have throughout the day to fill in the gaps. Snacks can contain those macronutrients you find challenging to include in meals.

3. *Ensure your meals contain the right balance:* When you're planning meals, check meal composition boxes to ensure your meals are balanced (protein, fat, and carbohydrate other than fruits and veggies).

4. *Don't skip breakfast:* If there is one meal that endurance athletes struggle with the most, it is breakfast. Whether it's a lack of appetite or planning that leads you to skip breakfast, it's essential to start your day off right

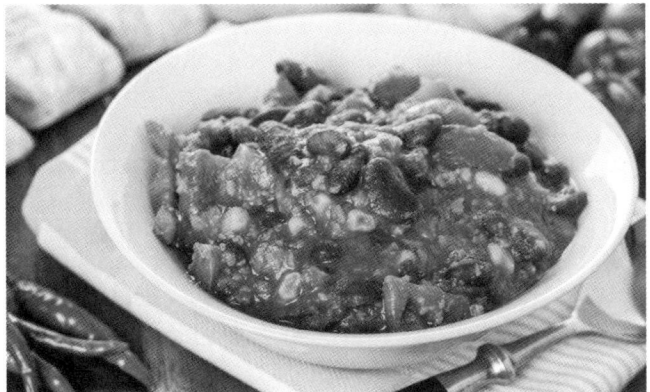

vertmedia/Getty Images/iStockphoto

Chilis can provide a balanced meal at lunch with little prep time.

with some fuel. If you really can't get much in, focus on smoothies or yogurt parfaits, which can allow you to sip slowly or eat a smaller, nutrient-packed food at your own pace.

5. *Pack your lunch:* Bringing your own nutrition to the office or even your at-home desk can lead to the best intentional choices to ensure you are getting everything you need. Think about easy options such as wraps, sandwiches, bowls, or chilis that provide a balanced meal with little prep.

Planning and Shopping Tips

The planning and shopping process doesn't have to be hard unless you make it hard. Benefits of planning meals and snacks ahead of time include the following:

- Less worry about what to fuel with during the work week
- Less stress and fatigue when deciding what to eat
- Less food waste, which is better for the environment
- Better energy levels and lower risk of underfueling
- Better performance and recovery

Often, endurance athletes make the following mistakes during the meal planning, shopping, and prepping process:

- *Too much repetition:* Having the same meals and snacks over and over can lead to boredom and palate fatigue—not to mention that decreased food diversity leads to less micronutrient intake.
- *Too complex:* Searching for recipes that require a lot of ingredients and prep time is usually overwhelming and not realistic for endurance athletes to maintain.
- *Trying to make everything from scratch:* Convenience items have their place, and having some backup items on hand in case you don't want to cook is crucial. Also, foods such as frozen fruits and veggies and microwavable rice or pasta can be time-saving options if you need the help.

To succeed with your nutrition, a little bit of structure is vital. Try to carve out a block of time to plan and shop. When deciding the best times for these important tasks, consider the following:

- *Don't rely on weekends:* This might not be the best time to plan, especially if you travel or do a lot of your training on the weekend, because your fatigue levels may be high.
- *Take advantage of rest days:* Rest days might be good days to plan because of the extra time you have when not training.

- *Create a recurring time block on your calendar each week:* A recurring time block can offer consistency and help you maintain a routine. A lunch hour or postwork block often works best.
- *Inventory your pantry:* Doing a biweekly or monthly inventory of your pantry can not only help you stay organized but also ensure you have key staples you might need throughout the week (see the Endurance Athlete Pantry Checklist later in this chapter).
- *Create a shopping routine:* If going to the store to pick out items isn't your thing, think about doing an online grocery order so you can shop from home and pick it up later. This can also prevent unnecessary spending. If you do like to frequent the grocery store, try to have a set day or days that you go.

Pantry Staples

Stocking your pantry with your favorite convenient options can help when you need to add a quick macronutrient to make a more balanced meal or snack or when you forget to go to the grocery store and just need to throw a meal together. The following are some of my favorite pantry staples that can help you stay prepared:

- *Dry oats:* Whether used as a prerun oatmeal snack (quick oats only due to lower fiber content, unless you want to find the nearest bathroom), an addition to smoothies, or for homemade granola, oats are a versatile pantry item that can help you reach your carb needs.
- *Granola:* Some granolas can be complete nutrition sources if they contain nuts, seeds, and dried fruit (protein, carboydrate, and fat). This can be helpful for athletes who need an easy way to get in more overall nutrition to support their training.
- *Dried fruit:* Dried fruit is a convenient, portable carb option that can be great by itself or as an addition to oatmeal or trail mix. Be cautious of sulfur dioxide, which is used as a preservative, because it may cause dizziness and headaches in those who are sensitive to it.
- *Precooked grains:* If you've tried to cook a perfect batch of rice or grain before, you know it can be tricky and time-consuming to get the right texture. This is where keeping frozen or shelf-stable precooked grains can come in handy. Pop them in the microwave or cook them on the stove to have carbs ready to add to any meal in moments.
- *Frozen waffles:* A convenient prerun option, frozen waffles pack in a lot of carbs.
- *Shelf-stable tofu:* Tofu is a plant-based protein option that can be used in smoothies, stir-fries, scrambles, and wraps; it can be tossed in just about anything to increase the protein content. Make sure

you keep a variety of textures in your pantry—silken to firm—to increase the versatility.

- *Shelf-stable nut milk:* Most commonly used as a smoothie base, nut milks can help you easily get in nutrition (carbs and protein) after a run. Choosing a nut milk that has protein in it (most contain a large percentage of water) is key. Aim for an option that has at least five to seven grams of protein per serving. If you are looking for some extra carbs, choose a sweetened variety.

- *Canned beans:* Great as an add-in to a meal or as the base of a stand-alone bean salad, canned beans are a great staple to get in extra carbs and protein. When choosing your beans, try to choose BPA-free cans to avoid possible health risks such as increased blood pressure and cardiovascular disease.

- *Cans or packs of tuna or salmon:* A quick snack or addition to any meal, wild salmon and tuna packs provide you with the protein you need and bonus omega-3 fatty acids with inflammation-balancing properties.

- *Chickpea pasta:* Complete with both carbs and protein, chickpea pasta (such as Banza pasta) can be a good base for meals or side dishes.

- *Protein powder:* While a food-first approach is always preferred, it can be helpful to have protein powder available to make a quick shake, increase the nutrition in your overnight oats, or even add a boost to your soup.

- *Olive or avocado oil:* Used as a dressing, sauce, or cooking base, olive and avocado oils contain inflammation-balancing mono- and polyunsaturated fatty acids.

- *Nut and seed butters:* A perfect addition to a meal or snack, nut and seed butters have a lot of nutrition with their fat and protein combo. Look out for added sugars and preservatives.

- *Jarred pesto:* Having a good pesto on hand can not only provide inflammation-balancing fats but also pack a lot of flavor into a meal.

- *Frozen fruits and vegetables:* It's always good to add some color to your meals and snacks to get the added antioxidants, vitamins, minerals, and fiber that fruits and vegetables provide. Try to choose a variety of colors to increase the diversity of your micronutrient intake and keep you healthy and running strong. Keep in mind that frozen fruits and vegetables are frozen at peak ripeness and keep much longer than their fresh counterparts.

To simplify the process and decide on some favorite pantry items to have available, you can use the following Endurance Athlete Pantry Checklist as a guide to help you do your inventory and create your shopping list. You don't need to have everything on the checklist on hand.

Endurance Athlete Pantry Checklist

Beans (Dried or Canned)
- ☐ Chickpeas
- ☐ Cannellini beans
- ☐ Black beans
- ☐ Kidney beans
- ☐ Pinto beans
- ☐ Lentils (green or red)

Spices and Herbs
- ☐ Salt
- ☐ Pepper
- ☐ Cinnamon
- ☐ Vanilla
- ☐ Dill
- ☐ Garlic
- ☐ Taco seasoning
- ☐ Oregano
- ☐ Rosemary
- ☐ Curry
- ☐ Turmeric
- ☐ Chili flakes

Grains
- ☐ Rice or wild rice
- ☐ Pasta
- ☐ Bread
- ☐ Tortillas
- ☐ Israeli couscous
- ☐ Farro
- ☐ Quinoa
- ☐ Oats
- ☐ Popcorn
- ☐ Breadcrumbs

Nuts and Seeds
- ☐ Walnuts
- ☐ Almonds
- ☐ Cashews
- ☐ Pistachios
- ☐ Chia seeds
- ☐ Ground flaxseed
- ☐ Sunflower seeds
- ☐ Pumpkin seeds
- ☐ Pine nuts

Nut and Seed Butters
- ☐ Peanut butter
- ☐ Almond butter
- ☐ Cashew butter
- ☐ Tahini
- ☐ Sunflower seed butter

Baking Essentials
- ☐ Flour
- ☐ Chocolate chips
- ☐ Baking powder
- ☐ Baking soda
- ☐ Sugar
- ☐ Brown sugar
- ☐ Corn bread mix
- ☐ Coconut flakes
- ☐ Maple syrup

Milks
- ☐ Almond milk
- ☐ Soy milk
- ☐ Oat milk
- ☐ Cow's milk
- ☐ Creamer
- ☐ Canned coconut milk

Vinegars
☐ Red wine vinegar   ☐ Rice vinegar
☐ Balsamic vinegar

Broths
☐ Vegetable broth   ☐ Beef broth
☐ Chicken broth

Oils
☐ Olive oil   ☐ Sesame oil
☐ Coconut oil   ☐ Ghee
☐ Avocado oil

Canned Vegetables and Fruits
☐ Tomatoes (crushed, whole,   ☐ Roasted red peppers
  chopped, and pureed)   ☐ Artichoke hearts
☐ Tomato sauce or paste   ☐ Olives
☐ Sun-dried tomatoes   ☐ Canned chilis

Frozen Vegetables and Fruits
☐ Broccoli   ☐ Shredded potatoes
☐ Cauliflower   ☐ Bell pepper mix
☐ Shelled edamame   ☐ Diced onions
☐ Corn   ☐ Mango
☐ Peas   ☐ Pineapple
☐ Green beans   ☐ Mixed berries
☐ Stir-fry mix   ☐ Tropical fruit mix
☐ Spinach

Condiments and Sauces
☐ Ketchup   ☐ Green curry paste
☐ Soy sauce or tamari   ☐ Red curry paste
☐ Dijon mustard   ☐ Pesto
☐ Mayonnaise   ☐ Salsa
☐ Stir-fry sauce

Proteins
☐ Shelf-stable tofu   ☐ Canned tuna
☐ Frozen shrimp   ☐ Frozen veggie burgers
☐ Frozen chicken breasts   ☐ Frozen ground meat

From K. Van Horn, *Practical Fueling for Endurance Athletes: Your Nutrition Guide for Optimal Performance,* (Champaign, IL: Human Kinetics, 2026).

Meal Planning

For endurance athletes with packed schedules, it can be hard to shop and cook every meal with fresh ingredients, get balanced nutrition, and ensure you are fueling enough. With limited hours in the day and many of us on a budget, time- and money-savers, such as meal planning, can help you fuel and reduce added pressures to have the perfect diet. Here are some helpful tips to optimize your meal planning:

1. *Cook once, eat twice (or multiple times):* If you don't have time to cook, batch-cooking a larger portion of food and eating it for multiple meals can help. Prepared food can typically be stored in the refrigerator for three to five days or frozen for one to two months. This option is best for those who don't want or need a lot of variety in their diet.

2. *Plan your pantry:* Think about dividing your pantry into different food categories that are freezable or shelf-stable (proteins, carbohydrates, fats, fruits and vegetables). List items in your pantry for each category and create a balanced meal plan, checking that each meal's composition categories will get you through two to three days in case you travel. For example, a balanced breakfast from the pantry could include protein-packed overnight oats—oats for carbohydrates, frozen berries for fruit, protein powder for protein, and peanut butter for fat. (Refer to the meal planning sheet later in this chapter.)

3. *Keep it simple:* Having too much variety in a weekly meal plan can lead to stress and burnout. Keep it simple by planning out one to two breakfasts, one to two lunches, three to five snacks, and three to four dinners so you have a little variety but aren't overwhelmed.

4. *Figure out how many nights you can realistically cook:* If you know you can't cook every night, that's OK. Just determine how many nights you can cook and then plan from there. Consider all your weekly commitments, and don't forget to include travel. Be sure to account for potentially tight time blocks when you might need quicker options.

- Early-morning workouts might require different preworkout snacks or quick postworkout meals if time is tight to get to work.
- Picking up the kids after your workout and then having dinner before soccer practice might require a prepared or convenience option.
- Double days of training offer their own unique challenges and may require lower-fiber options that are easier to grab.

5. *Use your plan to build your grocery list:* Once you simplify and plan your meals and snacks, do a quick inventory of what you already have, then make a list of what you need to get.

6. *Organize your shopping list by the store sections:* If you have a grocery store you shop at frequently, organize your shopping list by the store's sections to make the experience quicker and easier.

Exercise: Meal Planning From Your Pantry

Being prepared and having a backup meal plan that you can build directly from your freezer and pantry can benefit you greatly if you are traveling or if you simply couldn't make your weekly shopping trip. Complete this pantry meal and snack planning exercise to be prepared to fuel in case you find yourself in a bind.

Step One

Fill in each section with at least two items per category.

Proteins:

Carbohydrates:

Fats:

Fruits and vegetables:

Step Two

Create ideas for three breakfasts, three lunches, three snacks, and three dinners as backups if you can't shop. Use items from each meal composition category when building meals, and create balanced snack items with at least two macronutrients.

Breakfast:

1.

2.

3.

Lunch:

1.

2.

3.

Dinner:

1.

2.

3.

Snacks:

1.

2.

3.

From K. Van Horn, *Practical Fueling for Endurance Athletes: Your Nutrition Guide for Optimal Performance,* (Champaign, IL: Human Kinetics, 2026).

7. *Consider frozen food options:* Frozen meals, rice, vegetables, and fruit are often written off or forbidden because they are deemed unhealthy or inferior in some way. However, these items can save tons of time and can be repurposed as the base of a meal and then bulked up to fit your nutrition needs.

The following Meal Planning Sheet can be used to simplify your weekly meal and snack planning. The sheet allows for variety and purposefully does not assign meals and snacks to days of the week. Feel free to plan as few or as many as you want depending on how much variety you need in your eating pattern.

Meal Planning Sheet

Breakfast
1.
2.
3.

Lunch
1.
2.
3.

Dinner
1.
2.
3.
4.

Snacks
1.
2.
3.
4.
5.

Sometimes as a busy endurance athlete, you need some quick, balanced breakfasts and lunches to get you through your day that take less than 10 minutes to prepare. The following time-saving meals will help you meet your nutrition needs and stay satisfied.

Quick Breakfast Ideas
1. Overnight oats with protein powder, nut butter, jam, and berries
2. Greek yogurt with granola and strawberries

3. Toast with hummus; smashed hard-boiled eggs; apple
4. Egg-white wrap with veggies and avocado
5. Toast with peanut butter, Nutella, and sliced banana; glass of soy milk
6. Quick-cook oatmeal with sliced almonds, yogurt, nut butter, and blueberries
7. Frozen protein waffles with nut butter, syrup, and sliced banana
8. Chia seed pudding made with chia seeds, protein powder, almond milk, and blueberries
9. Smashed avocado and hard-boiled eggs on toast; grapes
10. Bagel with cream cheese; smoked salmon; banana

Packable Lunch Ideas

1. Tuna salad sandwich; apple slices
2. Turkey wrap with hummus, veggies, and cheese; grapes
3. Nut butter and jelly sandwich; yogurt with berries
4. Rice bowl with tofu, roasted veggies, dressing, and edamame
5. Salad with chicken, feta, dressing, and veggies; orange; crackers
6. Turkey and cheese rollup; crackers; hummus and veggies
7. Chicken pasta salad with veggies; cheese stick; handful of nuts
8. Pita with falafel, roasted veggies, and hummus; banana
9. Egg salad sandwich; veggies and pretzels with dip
10. Chili (regular or vegan) packed in a thermos; tortilla chips; apple

From K. Van Horn, *Practical Fueling for Endurance Athletes: Your Nutrition Guide for Optimal Performance,* (Champaign, IL: Human Kinetics, 2026).

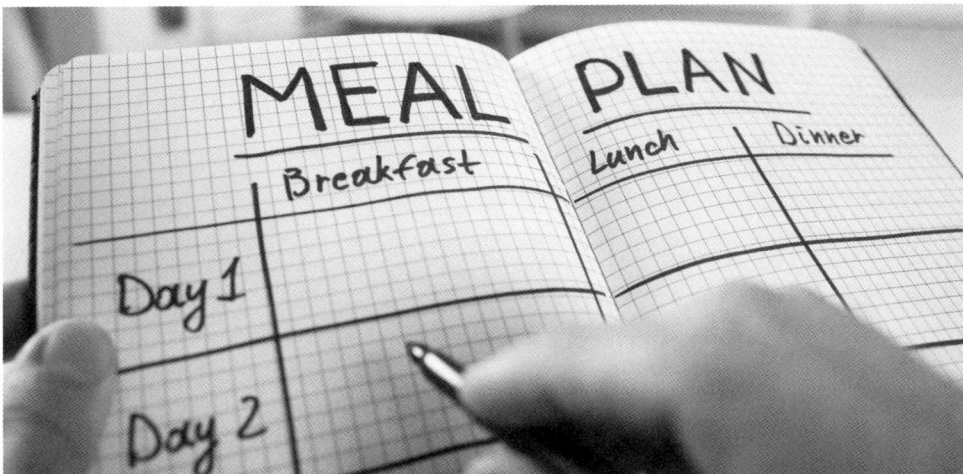

AndreyPopov/iStockphoto/Getty Images

Use a meal planning journal or the provided Meal Planning Sheet to plan out your meals each week.

Snack Planning

Many endurance athletes don't take the time to plan intentional snacks for themselves for the week. Framing snacks as a vehicle for added nutrition is a good way to view them because they can provide vital micro- and macronutrients to meet your needs. When planning intentional snacks, think about including one of each of the following types. Please use these as a starting point—you may need to adjust due to your preferences and needs.

Preworkout Snack

Before a workout, you want to give your body some fuel that is easy to digest without a lot of protein and fat. Emphasize simple carbohydrates (one to two grams per kilogram of body weight). Protein and fat, due to their slower digestion, should be limited to 10 to 15 grams each. It is important to test out different preworkout snacks because some athletes may need to include a little bit of protein and fat to prevent rebound hypoglycemia (a quick spike and drop in blood sugar).

Guidelines for Preworkout Snacks

Calories: 300 to 700

Carbohydrate: At least 1 to 2 grams per kilogram of body weight

Protein: 10 to 15 grams max

Fat: 10 to 15 grams max

Preworkout Snack Ideas

- Two frozen waffles with maple syrup
- Toast with nut butter; banana
- Dry cereal with a small amount of milk
- Graham crackers with fruit and honey
- Two pieces of toast with jam or jelly
- Fruit; granola bar
- Muffin; fruit
- Dates; nut butter
- Quick cook oats with honey
- Small bagel with cream cheese
- Toaster pastry

Spiced Sweet Potato Muffins

Full of carbs and a little bit of protein, these muffins are great for a preworkout snack or a tasty midday energy boost.

Ingredients

- 2 large eggs (substitute 1/4 cup [60 mL] Just Egg for vegans)
- 1 cup (230 g) mashed sweet potato
- 1/2 cup (120 mL) oil (avocado or olive oil work great)
- 1/4 cup (85 g) blackstrap molasses
- 1 tbsp ube extract (purple sweet potato extract)
- 1/2 cup (120 mL) water, oat milk, nut milk, or coconut milk
- 2 tbsp orange juice
- 1/4 tsp ground cloves
- 3/4 cup (90 g) mix of seeds (we use a chia, sunflower, pumpkin, and hemp combo)
- 1-2/3 cup (217 g) all-purpose flour
- 1-1/4 cup (250 g) sugar
- 1 tsp baking soda
- 1 tsp ground cinnamon
- 3/4 tsp salt
- 1/2 tsp baking powder
- 1/2 tsp ground nutmeg

Directions

1. Preheat oven to 350 °F (177 °C).
2. Whisk together eggs, mashed sweet potato, oil, molasses, ube extract, orange juice, and liquid choice (water, oat milk, nut milk, or coconut milk).
3. Add dry ingredients and mix until just combined. Overmixing may cause muffins to be rubbery or tough.
4. Pour into a greased 9 x 5 in. (27 x 15 cm) loaf pan or lined muffin pan.
5. Garnish the top with seeds or oats if desired.
6. Bake until the top is firm and set, about 25-30 minutes.
7. Cool and enjoy! It can be frozen for up to one month.

Postworkout Snack

The main purpose of a postworkout snack is to aid in muscle recovery and glycogen replenishment, so you'll want to refuel with some carbohydrate and protein. Emphasizing simple carbohydrates again will allow for the quickest glycogen replenishment rates. Ideal protein intake ranges from 20 to 30 grams, focusing on high BCAA sources.

Guidelines for Postworkout Snacks
Calories: 240 to 340
Carbohydrate: 1 to 4 grams per kilogram of body weight
Protein: At least 20 grams (high BCAA)

Postworkout Snack Ideas
- Protein shake; fruit
- Hard boiled eggs; dried fruit
- PB&J sandwich; yogurt
- Almonds; orange
- Yogurt with dried fruit and nuts
- Chocolate milk; banana
- Canned tuna with crackers
- Dry roasted edamame; fruit
- Avocado toast with eggs
- Cookies; protein shake

Everyday Snack

Planning and choosing snacks that are sufficient in size and balanced with two macronutrients can help the blood sugar stay stable and keep your energy high throughout the day. Everyday snacks can be as simple as combining two items together (such as an apple and nut butter) or as complex as you would like (high-protein energy bites). Ensuring variety in your sweet and savory choices for everyday snacks can keep you from getting tired of the same thing.

Guidelines for Everyday Snacks
Protein and carbohydrate
Protein and fat
Carbohydrate and fat

Everyday Snack Ideas
- Apple with nut or seed butter
- Trail mix
- Cottage cheese; bell peppers
- Popcorn; nuts
- Beef jerky; fruit
- Carrot or celery sticks with dressing or hummus
- Rollup with two slices of turkey deli meat and cheese
- Pretzels with nut butter
- Two slices of banana bread; nut butter
- Chia seed pudding

Bedtime Snack

A snack before bed can be helpful if you are trying to recover from high-intensity or heavier training days. When composing your bedtime snack, lean toward a high-protein option to increase muscle protein synthesis before sleep. Studies on snacking before bed have demonstrated that 30 grams of high-quality protein can increase muscle protein synthesis rates while sleeping (Snijders et al. 2019).

Guidelines for Bedtime Snacks

Calories: 200 to 300

Protein: 30 grams

Carbohydrate: less than 30 grams

Bedtime Snack Ideas

- 1 cup (230 g) Greek yogurt with berries and granola
- 1 oz (30 g) cheese and crackers
- Half a protein smoothie
- 1/4 cup (30 g) trail mix; 8 oz (240 mL) milk
- Hard-boiled egg; 1/4 cup (30 g) almonds
- 1 cup (230 g) cottage cheese; berries
- 1 cup (160 g) roasted chickpeas
- 1/2 cup (115 g) oatmeal (cooked); nut butter
- Two cheese sticks; berries
- Half a muffin; 8 oz (240 mL) milk

Peanut Butter Chocolate Chip Date Ball Recipe

This recipe makes a great bedtime snack.
Servings: 6 (2 balls per serving)

Ingredients

- 1 cup (175 g) pitted dates
- 1/4 cup (65 g) peanut butter
- 1/8 tsp sea salt
- 2 tbsp chocolate chips

Directions

1. Add dates to a food processor and blend.
2. Add peanut butter and salt to the date puree and blend until combined.
3. Add chocolate chips and pulse until incorporated.
4. Form into 1-in. balls and place on parchment paper or in container.
5. Freeze balls for at least an hour and store in refrigerator or freezer.

Raspberry Vanilla Chocolate Chip Chia Seed Pudding

A combination of high protein and a little bit of carbohydrate makes this pudding a great bedtime recovery snack.
Servings: 2

Ingredients

- 1/4 cup (40 g) chia seeds
- 1 cup (240 mL) unsweetened oat milk (almond, flax, or regular milk all work as well)
- 1/4 cup vanilla protein powder
- 3/4 cup (100 g) raspberries (divided)
- 2 tbsp unsweetened coconut flakes (optional)
- 2 tsp chocolate chips (optional)

Directions

1. In a large bowl, mix chia seeds, oat milk, and protein powder. Mix well so that all protein powder is thoroughly incorporated. Refrigerate for 20 minutes or overnight.
2. In a small bowl, smash up half the raspberries.
3. Top with smashed raspberries, remaining whole raspberries, chocolate chips, and coconut flakes.

Essential Kitchen Tools

Who doesn't like saving time while cooking? You can do just that with the right set of kitchen tools to fit your lifestyle, meal preparation, and batch-cooking habits. Kitchen tools may be intimidating if you have never used them before, but once you learn the necessary skills, they are very useful. Whether you are setting up your kitchen for the first time or wanting to optimize what you have available, here are some of my favorite options to make cooking quicker and more enjoyable:

- *Rice cooker:* Batch-cook grains to use throughout the week to meet carbohydrate requirements for different training days.
- *Instant Pot:* An Instant Pot can double as a slow cooker or rice cooker. Use it to make a quick, large batch of food you can eat throughout the week.
- *Blender:* Particularly useful when you lack an appetite after a workout, a blender can help you whip up a high-calorie smoothie to sip on to get all your nutrients in.
- *Mandoline:* This underrated kitchen tool can save you a significant amount of time chopping and prepping veggies for the week.

- *Immersion blender:* An immersion, or stick, blender can help when you just need a quick blend or want to make a soup without having to dirty all the traditional blender parts.
- *Baking sheet(s):* For quick meal options with easy cleanup, baking sheets are wonderful. They're great for weekly meal prep or an entire meal.

Three Ways to Repurpose and Use Leftovers

1. *Blend it:* Blend up any fruit that is about to turn bad, or cut it up for a smoothie bowl.
2. *Make it a bowl:* Combine leftovers into a layered bowl option. Add a sauce or dressing to the top to give it some extra flavor.
3. *Roll it up:* You can put anything into a tortilla, right? Place leftovers into a tortilla and roll it up for a quick breakfast, lunch, or dinner.

Consider the Environment

On the surface, becoming a more environmentally conscious endurance athlete might seem a little overwhelming, especially with the discussions around all the things you "should" do to become a more sustainable version of yourself. Sustainability is not always an area of focus for endurance athletes when it comes to nutrition. However, choosing small ways to contribute to the future of our planet can add up in a big way, especially when you are working on your planning, shopping, and fueling habits.

1. *Make your own sports nutrition products or buy from sports nutrition companies that are trying to reduce their environmental impact.*

Finding eco-friendly sports nutrition products can be challenging. When you think about the number of prepackaged options you use on a yearly basis, the waste can add up.

Aim to reduce your fossil-fuel consumption and waste generation by cutting out plastic wrappers and packaging where you can. Do a quick online search to find refillable flasks or baby food pouches you can fill with maple syrup, honey, or (do-it-yourself) DIY food blend recipes (see the whole-food blend recipes in chapter 3). Carrying mini muffins or cookies in reusable silicone pouches or beeswax wrappers is an easy option.

If you don't have time or don't want to make your own food at home, the next best thing is to choose companies that are reducing their environmental impact or are committed to supporting the environment. Clif Bar and Company is part of the Ellen MacArthur Foundation Global

Commitment, which pledges to help create a world where plastic never becomes waste or pollution. They are committed to creating more eco-friendly packaging and driving education by using the How2Recycle label on their packaging. Other brands like GU Energy Labs are doing their part by improving their production process. They produce 95 percent of their energy needs from solar panels installed at their headquarters, use nontoxic cleaning products, and have reduced their water usage by 20 percent. Is it perfect? No, but it's a start.

2. *Buy locally or in season.*

Purchasing locally grown or in-season produce can support not only soil health and the environment but also local small businesses. Small-scale local farming can maximize soil health by increasing crop diversity, rotating crops, and ensuring regular soil fertilization. Maximizing soil health allows the soil to absorb more water and retain more carbon. As a bonus, purchasing locally lets you eat seasonal produce items, which are fresher and more nutritious due to the shorter time between harvest and consumption.

Purchasing produce from community-supported agriculture (CSA) programs and farmers markets helps farmers capture a higher profit margin. As part of a CSA program, you pay a fee that covers the costs of farming and harvesting. In exchange, you receive a box of local produce each week. To find a CSA program near you, you can use the USDA's CSA Directory.

3. *Inventory and plan.*

When you set aside time to plan and inventory every week, you can save money at the grocery store and help the environment by not overbuying food. Make sure you inventory what you have in the fridge, freezer, and pantry. If you have to use foods up, try to repurpose them into a new, creative meal. If you have foods that you know are going to spoil, preserve them in the freezer until you have time to use them.

Ways to Avoid Food Waste

While it is very difficult to eliminate all food waste, taking small steps to use foods that are getting ready to spoil can minimize the amount you throw away each week. Apply the following tips to help you on your own food-waste journey:

1. Blend up veggies, pour them into muffin tins, and freeze them to use in soups, sauces, and stews in the future.

2. Blanching and freezing veggies in bags can keep them good for weeks.

3. Grind up fresh herbs and freeze them in ice cube trays to make pesto.

4. Combine overripe berries with sugar and lemon juice and cook for 15 to 20 minutes over medium heat to make a jam.

5. Peel and chop up bananas and put them in reusable bags in the freezer to use in smoothies.

6. Keep the trimmings from broccoli, carrots, onions, asparagus, and peppers in a plastic bag in the freezer. Use them in soups and stocks when needed.

You can also keep your produce fresh longer by following these tips:

1. *Onions and garlic:* Store in a dark, cool place.

2. *Potatoes:* Store in a dark, cool place away from onions and garlic.

3. *Berries:* Do not wash until you are ready to eat.

4. *Avocados:* Ripen on the counter. Once they are ripe, store them in the refrigerator.

5. *Tomatoes:* Store in a bowl away from direct sunlight.

6. *Citrus fruits:* Store in the refrigerator for two weeks or on the counter for one week.

7. *Leafy greens:* Either wash, dry, and store in a sealed container lined with paper towels or store unwashed in a container or reusable bag.

8. *Apples:* Store in the refrigerator in a sealed bag.

Compost

One of the easiest ways to reduce your environmental footprint is to compost. According to the Environmental Protection Agency (EPA), composting can help sequester carbon and reduce greenhouse gases on a larger scale. Home composting can be done in even the smallest of spaces and can repurpose kitchen scraps for soil, which keeps them out of landfills, where they contribute to increased methane production.

To get started with composting, you can buy an official container or simply use a cardboard box. Composting a mix of greens (e.g., food scraps, coffee), browns (e.g., dead leaves, branches), and a little bit of water can ensure you have the right mix of carbon, nitrogen, and moisture to encourage your compost to thrive. Once it's ready, you can use it in your home garden, fertilize houseplants with it, donate it to a school or community garden, or take it to a local farmers market that gives the option to bring your compost.

Takeaways

- As an endurance athlete, you can take all the necessary steps to optimize your race fueling, but without foundational daily fueling practices, you'll never be able to reach your maximum potential.

- Intentional or unintentional shortages in nutrition can inhibit training adaptations, delay recovery, and increase your risk of illness and injury.

- Learning how to plan and prepare to fuel yourself properly should be the first step in this process before you make smaller tweaks to your diet to enhance your health and performance.

- When thinking about your own daily nutrition, review this chapter to ensure you understand the whats and whys before working on the hows.

- Remember that every endurance athlete is an individual; take care to figure out what will work best for you in the long run.

- While meal planning, prepping, and shopping might seem stressful, they don't have to be.

PART II

NUTRIENT TIMING STRATEGIES

8

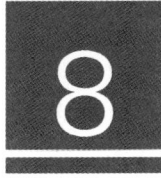

PREWORKOUT AND PRERACE FUELING

Back when I was a marathoner, I worked with a dietitian and learned about sodium preloading strategies and eating simple carbs to do a carb increase before big events. I credit focusing on my prerace and race nutrition strategies [for] helping me transition to my 50-mile world record.

—Camille Herron, professional ultra runner and world record holder in multiple ultra distances (athlete interview, 2022)

In order to capitalize on workout and race performances, most endurance athletes understand that an intraworkout fueling plan is important. However, they often overlook preworkout and prerace fueling, which could make or break performance goals on race day. Choose the wrong options, and you'll end up running for the nearest bushes—or worse, doubled over and forced to take a did not finish (DNF). Choose options that work for and with you, and you could end up with your next personal record (PR).

Pretraining and prerace fueling strategies include being intentional with fluid, electrolyte, and calorie choices. In certain instances, your choices multiple days before key workouts and training will have an impact. The following strategies will help you build a preworkout and prerace fueling strategy that is optimal for you and your sport-specific goals.

Pretraining Meal or Snack

Before any activity over 60 minutes, it's a good idea to fill up your fuel tank, especially if it is a morning training session after a night of sleep. Think of the pretraining meal or snack as your insurance policy to help you get through your training session and meet your racing goals.

To Snack or Not to Snack, That Is the Question

When doing a training session of less than an hour, many endurance athletes struggle with the question of whether they should fuel. In practice, I see a lot of endurance athletes who end up unintentionally underfueling, so I usually advise to err on the side of caution and have a snack. But if you would like to have a bit more nuance and context, you can ask yourself the following questions:

1. *How long has it been since my last snack or meal?* If it has been at least three to four hours, it is likely time to have a snack.

2. *Am I hungry?* If you're hungry, respond to those hunger cues and have a snack.

3. *Did I just wake up from a night of sleep?* You might want to have a snack even before shorter training sessions in the morning.

4. *Why?* Because cortisol levels are higher in the morning, and exercising without a snack or meal can raise those levels even more. This is particularly important for endurance athletes who are prone to injuries.

The goals of the pretraining meal or snack are to

1. fill glycogen stores and prolong carb stores for a session,
2. ensure proper hydration, and
3. prevent hunger and hypoglycemia (low blood sugar).

When considering options that might work best for you, take into account the following guidelines for calories, macronutrients, timing, and hydration.

Calories

Caloric intake before exercise ensures that you have enough fuel to keep you going throughout your entire training session. Hello, stable energy levels! For some endurance athletes, fueling before a session can seem like a chore, especially when training in the early hours of the day when appetite may be low. This is why it is important to discover what might work for you at different times of the day and have options to go along with your training schedule.

Caloric Intake for Training Sessions of Less Than Two Hours: 200 to 500

Examples of preworkout or prerace snacks and meals include the following:

- Banana with 1 tbsp peanut butter
- Bagel with 2 tbsp jam
- Granola bar and a banana
- Four graham crackers with 1 tbsp peanut butter (great for early-morning sessions)
- 10 oz (300 mL) of sports drink and 1 to 2 gels (great for early-morning sessions)
- Two squeezable fruit pouches such as from Noka (great for early-morning sessions)

Caloric Intake for Training Sessions of More Than Two Hours: 500 to 700

Examples of preworkout or prerace snacks and meals include the following:

- Bagel with 2 tbsp peanut butter, banana, 1/4 cup (60 g) granola, and 1 tbsp honey
- Two frozen waffles with 1 tbsp peanut butter, 2 tbsp syrup, and a banana
- Lärabar, a banana, 1 tbsp peanut butter, and 17 oz (510 mL) of sports drink with high-carbohydrate mix

Carbohydrate

Preexercise carbohydrate needs vary, but targets should be between 0.5 and 2.0 grams per kilogram of body weight. Aim to keep fiber to a minimum; a good guideline is less than five grams total. Avoid multigrain products, brown rice, beans, fruit, and whole rolled oats if you have a sensitive stomach because the fiber can be tougher for your digestive system to process. Most of your preexercise fuel should be composed of simple carbohydrates like white bread, honey, maple syrup, frozen waffles, pastries, muffins, and white bagels to reduce the chances of gastrointestinal distress.

Fat

Fat tolerance can vary depending on the athlete, but in general, because fats are digested much slower, use caution with the total amount you consume before exercise. No more than 5 to 10 grams is a good target.

Protein

Including some protein (8 to 15 grams) in your preexercise fuel can slow the release of carbohydrates into the bloodstream. This decreases the chance of rebound hypoglycemia, the abrupt drop in blood sugar that leads to energy highs and lows once your carbohydrate stores are burned up. Keep in mind that protein is digested slower, so too much can cause stomach sloshing, pain, or bathroom urgency.

Timing

The timing of your preexercise meal depends on your tolerance. Giving yourself time to digest can prevent cramping and allow your body to use the food you ate. It is always a good idea to practice with different options before making your final decision (such as during a long training session leading up to a goal race). Try to err on the side of caution and give yourself one to three hours to digest your preexercise fuel. If you are short on time (less than an hour before the training session), grab a quick carb-rich snack that has about 200 to 300 calories, such as dry cereal, a granola bar, or some graham crackers, to ensure quicker digestion and some energy to fuel your session.

Hydration

For many endurance athletes, it can be hard to keep up with hydration requirements during exercise; therefore, hydrating before a workout is key to starting the training session off right. While you can drink water and electrolytes according to thirst before exercise, try to avoid taking in straight fluids (sans electrolytes) because this may cause excessive urination.

Using a preexercise hyperhydration strategy has been shown to improve exercise capacity by reducing the heart rate and core body temperature. You can use chloride or sodium citrate, which may be slightly more palatable, as agents to draw fluids into the body and retain them because consuming these agents with fluids decreases urine output.

To perform an intentional hyperhydration strategy, consume 1,000 to 2,000 milligrams of sodium in 16 to 20 ounces (480 to 600 mL) of fluids two hours before exercise. Some companies make products formulated as a hyperhydration formula, but you can try using miso soup or another type of broth as an alternative. Some endurance athletes may respond better to a night-before hyperhydration strategy instead of the morning of, which is why it's so important to test it before a target event.

A word of caution: Because of the sheer amount of sodium coming into the body, you should definitely test the hyperhydration strategy before a target event. For some individuals, this strategy can increase gastrointestinal distress or blood pressure. Those with preexisting health conditions should proceed with caution.

Troubleshooting Side Stitches: A Preworkout Fueling Problem?

You'll know side stitches when they hit. It's a sharp, stabbing pain below the rib cage that seemingly comes out of nowhere. The interesting thing about side stitches is that they typically don't have an exact cause but can stem from several different factors. Let's look at a few of the most common causes:

1. *Weak core muscles and biomechanical imbalances:* Whether you are riding, running, swimming, or hiking, strength imbalances can cause a lack of core stabilization, which leads to stitches.

   Solution: Work with a strength trainer, physical therapist (PT), or gait specialist to get imbalances under control.

2. *Breathing and oxygen imbalances:* Exercising at too fast of a pace and not taking deep breaths can prevent oxygen from being delivered to the working muscles and cause issues with the diaphragm, leading to side stitches.

   Solution: Work on breathing and pacing during exercise to help oxygenate the system.

3. *Preworkout or race nutrition:* The timing and composition of preworkout or prerace nutrition can cause side stitches due to decreased blood flow and gastric emptying when exercise starts.

   Solution: Evaluate your preexercise fueling strategy. Double-check that your preworkout or prerace nutrition contains less than five grams of fiber and less than 10 grams of protein and fat. Be sure that solid food is consumed one to three hours ahead of time. Hydration should be sipped on rather than gulped in large amounts. Consuming an electrolyte solution can encourage fluids to absorb into the system more efficiently rather than just sit in the stomach.

Prerace Fueling Strategies

What if you knew that prerace nutrition could improve your performance by up to 3 percent? Yes, you *could* get away with improvising your nutrition plan, but having an intentional race-week nutrition plan could make the difference between dragging yourself across the finish line or feeling your best on race day. In this section, you'll learn best practices and tips to help you peak for your event.

Race-Week Strategies for Shorter Events (Less Than 60 minutes)

If you are eating a balanced diet (yes, including carbohydrates), you likely do not need to gradually increase carbohydrate intake leading up to a shorter race. Your muscles and liver store enough carbohydrate to fuel you for 90 minutes to 2 hours of endurance activity before you run out of energy and need to slow your pace. However, if you are following any kind of low-carbohydrate diet or are not being intentional enough about replacing carbohydrates to support your training, you could risk depleting your glycogen stores during your race. Remember, to perform at a higher percentage of your $\dot{V}O_2$max (e.g., in a 5K or sprint triathlon), you need a high amount of carbohydrate to ensure you can hold your desired pace.

In the one to two days before your target race, pay attention to hydration, electrolytes, and filling up glycogen stores. During these days, try to focus on simple carbohydrate choices (white rice, bread, pasta, honey, and maple syrup) to keep your fiber intake low and your digestive system happy. As a note, you do *not* need to eat 10 plates of pasta the night before your event. This will likely just leave you feeling bloated and uncomfortable on the starting line. It can be a good idea to limit fruit and vegetable consumption to cooked or blended varieties only—nothing raw. Try to stick with foods that are bland and familiar to you. Now is not the time to be adventurous with your restaurant food choices, or you may find yourself in the bathroom a lot before or during the race.

Be sure to hydrate with more than just water, which may flush out your electrolytes and put you at risk of developing a condition called *hyponatremia* where your blood sodium gets too low. A good general principle to help you hydrate before your event is to alternate between an electrolyte drink and plain water each time you fill up a water bottle or glass.

Some Notes on Travel Nutrition

You've spent months or even years preparing for a big endurance event. Traveling to a new place with new foods can bring up fears about how you'll feel on race day. Bringing your own food or anticipating restaurant or food options ahead of time is a great way to ease your nerves and avoid food poisoning (especially if you are traveling to another country with different sanitation standards). The following are some tips to help you transition quickly and have you energized for race day.

• *Airplane travel hydration and nutrition:* If you're traveling to your destination on an airplane, the flight itself can be dehydrating because you are flying at high altitude. Sip on fluids and electrolytes throughout the flight to stay hydrated. Avoid drinking alcohol on the plane because this can make you feel worse and increase your dehydration. Pack your own snacks to ensure that you are taking in regular nutrition. Here are some examples of packable travel snacks to fuel you during your trip:

- Protein powder packets (you can quickly add these to nonperishable milks or water)
- Dried fruit
- Trail mix
- Granola bars and protein bars
- Quick-cook oatmeal packets
- Nut butter packets
- Jerky

• *Hotel room nutrition:* Plan some fueling options for your hotel room if you don't have access to a kitchen. If the room has a mini fridge and a microwave, that's a bonus! Here are some foods you can make in a hotel room:

- Canned soup
- Instant oatmeal
- Pancakes
- Tuna packs
- Precooked and prepackaged noodles or rice
- Frozen burritos
- Frozen meals
- Instant cup of noodles
- Protein bars and shakes
- Cereal and granola
- Yogurt

• *Out-of-country hydration and nutrition:* If you are traveling to a new country that poses higher risks of food and water contamination (Asia, the Middle East, South America, Africa, and parts of Europe), use caution around new foods and consider the following:

- Stick with bland, more familiar food that you know you can tolerate.
- Avoid fresh vegetables and fruits and only choose those that have a peel.
- Don't eat food from street carts until after your race.
- Don't drink tap water or use ice. Drink bottled water only.
- Bring a probiotic supplement and stomach medication such as Imodium or Tums.

The prerace meal for a shorter endurance event should still be sufficient to ensure you've got enough carbohydrate in your system, don't get hungry or experience low energy at the starting line, and are fully hydrated. Stick to one to four grams per kilogram of body weight for carbohydrate, and similar to what you should do during the entire prerace week, choose low-fiber, simple carbohydrates. Even if you are nervous or nauseated before the event, it is still advisable to consume *something* before the race. Use liquid options like juice, a smoothie, or a hydration mix that contains calories—but be sure you're drinking something familiar.

Whatever you consume, give yourself enough time to digest; otherwise, you could end up feeling overly full and uncomfortable. For most athletes, this time frame ranges anywhere from one to three hours before the race, but you really need to test this ahead of time in your training workouts to see what works best for you.

Sipping on your favorite electrolyte drink, sports drink, or juice can ensure you are fully hydrated when you get to the starting line. However, use caution with the amount of fluids you consume before the race so you don't have to stop within the first five minutes. Caffeine consumption is optional, but if you are used to having coffee or tea, don't skip it on race day, or you could end up with a headache and other unwanted side effects such as nausea and anxiety.

Race-Week Nutrition Strategies for Rowing

For most short endurance races, the race-week nutrition strategy is an abbreviated version of its longer counterparts. Rowing, on the other hand, is a unique endurance sport, and as a result, precompetition nutrition methods should reflect this.

> For the majority of rowers, the gun goes off, and the race is over in a mere six to eight minutes. This leaves very little time for fueling during the event. Emily Edison, sports dietitian at the University of Washington, says the biggest mistake that she sees with her rowers is not fueling enough throughout the day, which can lead to deficient glycogen stores and increased risk of bonking during racing (interview, December 2022).

Reprinted by permission of Emily Edison.

Rowing is a unique endurance sport that uses anaerobic and aerobic systems to power through race events. Rowers race either individually or as part of a team and can be classified as single, double or pair, four or quad, or eight-member teams. Rowing races are typically 2,000 meters long, which ranges from six to eight minutes. The race is divided into three phases: the start phase, the middle or distance phase, and the finish or sprint phase (FISA, the World Rowing Federation 2002). The middle or distance phase relies on aerobic metabolism for energy production, which is why rowing is classified as an endurance sport.

Because of the short duration of rowing races, nutrition outside that race window becomes increasingly important for the athlete's success. Going into a race underfueled can make the difference between winning and losing. Rowing relies on both the anaerobic and aerobic systems for energy production, so the majority of energy substrate depends on muscle and liver glycogen status (Kim and Kim 2020). There is a lack of nutrition studies and congruent information on recommendations for rowers, but there are some nutritional strategies that we do know affect performance on race day.

Rowing athletes train one to three times per day, five to six days per week, which means they have high energy demands and can easily deplete their glycogen stores. Overall energy intake must be sufficient to support their body and prevent overtraining. Daily carbohydrate demands range from 5 to 12 grams per kilogram of body weight per day. Because these races are short, rowers do not need to engage in a gradual carbohydrate increase to supersaturate their glycogen stores; however, if their regular, daily fueling is not optimized, they may enter competition without sufficient glycogen stores to push their performance limits in the race.

Dehydration can be detrimental to rowers if they are not replacing lost fluids daily. Fluid losses tend to be high due to heat and wind exposure out on the water. Because the sport tends to focus on an athlete's weight, rowers who are trying to "make weight" (achieve a certain weight) may struggle with hydration status as they cut down closer to the event. Remember that more than 2 percent loss in body weight from fluids can affect performance due to reduced blood flow and increased core body temperature (Kelly, Nepotiuk, and Brown 2021). Many rowers take dehydration to the extreme, so hydrating after weighing in with an electrolyte solution can help. However, trying to fully rehydrate within the two hours between the weigh-in and the start of the race can be quite difficult.

Weigh-ins for rowing events can complicate prerace nutrition strategies tremendously. Because athletes need to make weight, they may engage in extremely restrictive practices that can affect their overall performance in the race. It can be beneficial for rowers who need to make weight to think about attaining a more sustainable daily body weight instead of engaging in restrictive practices before races; this can reduce the impact on their race-day performance.

Race-Week Fueling
for Longer Endurance Events

Here we'll address your race-week fueling needs for longer events, including marathons, endurance cycling races, obstacle course racing (OCR) races, Ironman 70.3 and Ironman distances, and ultramarathons. For many long-distance endurance athletes, the phrase *carb load* brings up visions of overflowing plates of pasta and pizza the night before a race and memories of nausea and bathroom breaks. On average, the storage capacity for glycogen between the liver and muscles is about 1,800 to 2,000 calories, but depending on sex, body weight, training status, and diet, this can increase up to 3,200 calories. That provides enough fuel for 90 minutes to 2 hours of exercise before you "hit the wall" (reach physical exhaustion). Think of it this way: Supersaturating your glycogen stores before a longer event can ensure you have a full gas tank when you go into the event.

The idea of the carbohydrate load was first studied in the 1960s, when Scandinavian scientists had a group of cyclists bike to exhaustion and measured their muscle glycogen content. They compared the cyclists' performances when they had eaten a high-carb diet before their tests with their performances after a low-carb meal. On the high-carb diet, they were able to cycle three to four times longer, indicating there was something to this study (Bergström et al. 1967).

Carbohydrate loading was not truly put into practice until 1969, when British runner Ron Hill used the strategy as part of his training to win the gold medal in the marathon at the European Athletic Championships in Greece. At the time, Hill was the first one to try carbohydrate loading as a performance-enhancing strategy. Prior to his experimentation, no one had even heard of it. Using the strategy of depleting his glycogen stores by eating higher protein, followed by supersaturating his muscles with carbohydrates a few days before the marathon, he was able to avoid hitting the dreaded wall (Oliver 2019). From that point on, runners began to use carbohydrate loading for their own performance benefits, and a protocol developed: a few days of a lower carb, higher protein diet and higher intensity training followed by a few days of lower volume and higher carbohydrate intake. Eventually, this somehow evolved into endurance athletes eating heaps of pasta the day before a big race, which can open the door to stomach distress on race day.

More recent research on carbohydrate loading shows that endurance training and carb increases combine well when done properly. It turns out that our bodies are pretty good at carbohydrate loading in the three days before a target event without doing a higher intensity, lower carb depletion period. The combined effect of tapering (reducing training volume and intensity) and increasing carbohydrates in the days prior to an event is enough to fill up glycogen stores (Sherman et al. 1981).

How to Implement an Intentional Carbohydrate Increase

To get the most benefit from carbohydrate loading before a race, you need to do it correctly. Without proper insight into how much you really need, you may be missing out on your diet's full potential. While it may vary based on your current carbohydrate intake, a carbohydrate load can range from 5 to 12 grams per kilogram of body weight per day.

For a 150-pound endurance athlete, that means between 477 and 818 grams of total carbohydrate per day in the three to five days leading up to an event. Keep in mind that the sheer amount of carbohydrate can be difficult for even the most experienced runners to get in, so it's important to figure out what strategies work best for you. The goal isn't to approach the starting line bloated and nauseated.

Consider these tips when deciding on your carb strategy:

- *Choose simple carbohydrates:* Focus on simple carbohydrates because of their lower fiber content. They're often easier to eat, and the lower fiber can help prevent gastrointestinal distress during the run. Examples include pretzels, white rice, white pasta, juice, and bagels. Table 8.1 offers more suggestions.

- *Watch your fruit and vegetable intake:* Too much fiber from raw fruits and vegetables can lead to gastrointestinal distress. In general, keep your intake to less than 20 grams per day for the few days leading up to your target race to reduce stress on the system. However, this may be too low for some athletes, so a more gradual fiber taper might be best to prevent constipation.

- *Drink hydration mix:* This not only helps you meet your carbohydrate needs but also gives you a hydration and electrolyte boost, both of which are important before a race.

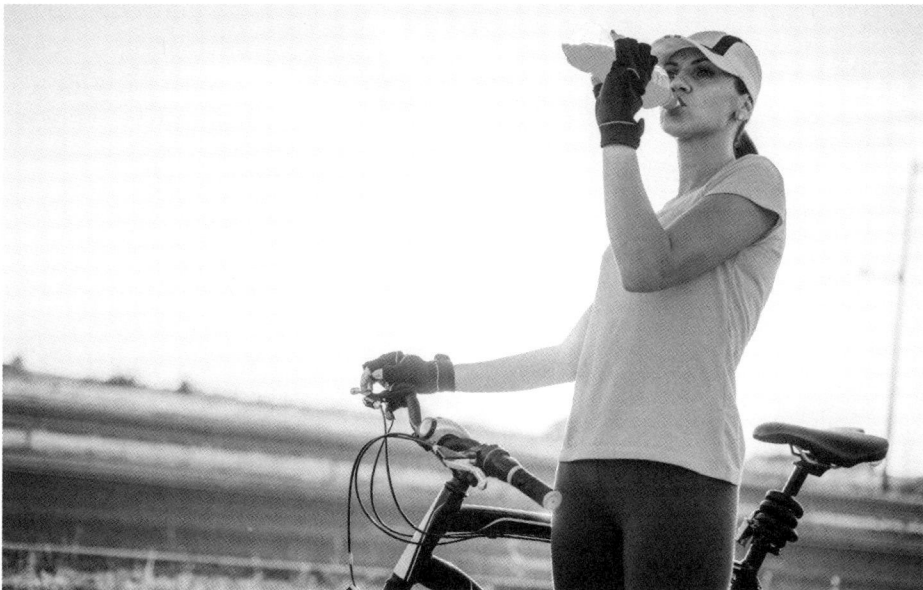

Drazen_/E+/Getty Images

Drinking hydration mix can help you meet your carbohydrate needs and give you a hydration and electrolyte boost.

- *Use snacks:* Spreading out your carbohydrates throughout the day and including carbohydrate-rich snacks can make it less intimidating than eating a huge pasta dinner the night before your race.
- *Plan ahead:* Know your snacking strategy and carb sources ahead of time. This will help you hit your targets without trying to figure it out spontaneously.
- *Reduce your protein and fat intake:* Protein and fat take longer to digest and fill you up quicker, making it harder to get enough carbs. You don't need to eliminate them completely, but replacing some of your fat or protein with carbs will make the carb load easier.

TABLE 8.1   Simple Carb-Rich Foods and Amount of Carbohydrate per Portion

Food type	Portion of food	Amount of carbohydrate per portion
Banana	1 medium	27 g
White bread	2 slices standard	45 g
White bagel	1 medium	53 g
White pasta	1 cup (160 g) cooked	45 g
White rice	1 cup (190 g) cooked	44 g
Mini pretzel twists	18 twists	44 g
Frozen waffles	1 waffle	30 g
Graham crackers	2 sheets	22 g
Swedish Fish	5 pieces	27 g
Potatoes	1 cup (160 g)	45 g
Chocolate chip cookies	1 cookie	20 g
Medjool dates	2 whole	36 g
Orange juice	8 oz (240 mL)	26 g
Honey	1 tbsp	15 g
Jam	1 tbsp	15 g
Ritz crackers	10 crackers	20 g
White pita bread	1 6-in. (15 cm) pita	30 g
Fruit snacks	1 pouch	20 g
Applesauce (sweetened)	1 package	17 g

High-Carbohydrate Snack Ideas

Having some reliable higher carbohydrate snacks can give endurance athletes options when traveling and also allow snacks to fill in the gaps if prerace nerves have taken over during the carbohydrate increase.

- Bagel with 2 tbsp jam
- Bowl of your favorite cereal with milk
- 4 graham crackers with nut or seed butter
- 4 dates stuffed with nut butter
- 4 to 5 Oreo cookies with milk
- 16 oz (480 mL) of juice or hydration mix
- 2 toaster pastries
- Handful of crackers with cheese
- Granola bar with 8 oz (240 mL) of juice
- Tortilla wrap with nut or seed butter

Prerace Meal

Plan on eating a carbohydrate-rich meal two to three hours before your race begins. Ideally, the meal will contain one to two grams of carbohydrate per kilogram of body weight and a little bit of fat and protein to bring your calorie total to about 500 to 700 calories. Skipping a prerace meal should never be an option, especially if this will be the first meal you have had in over 12 hours. Starting a longer endurance event in a fasted state is a recipe for disaster.

If prerace nerves get in the way of you being able to consume solid food, consider practicing with an all-liquid option such as a high-carbohydrate drink mix or smoothie in the training sessions leading up to your event. You can consume caffeine found in coffee and tea (three to six milligrams per kilogram of body weight) but remember, it is a gastrointestinal stimulant and can upset your stomach on race day if you use too much of it. Be sure to check the weather forecast and determine whether you will

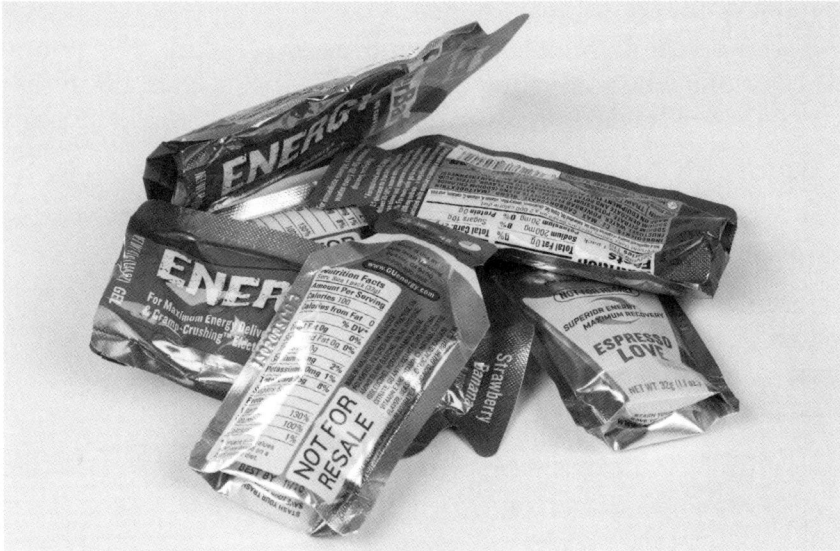

Energy gels can provide endurance athletes with a boost before and during their events, however, be sure to practice your fueling routine before event day to make sure it works for you.

need extra electrolytes because of excessive heat or humidity. In general, avoid drinking straight water so you don't flush out your electrolytes. Some athletes choose to take an energy gel 30 to 60 minutes before the gun goes off, but there is no scientific benefit to doing so—if it works for you, go for it! All in all, it is a good idea to practice your prerace meal before race day to ensure it will work for your gastrointestinal system.

Hydration Tip

In the days leading up to your race, be sure to hydrate with more than just water. Focusing on hydration is important in the lead-up to race day, but if you drink too much water, you risk flushing out your electrolytes. This can lead to a potentially life-threatening condition called hyponatremia (low blood sodium levels). To avoid this, sip on electrolytes with your fluids throughout the day in the one to three days leading up to the race.

The following are some prerace meal ideas. Again, be sure to test these during your training well before race day.

- 1 cup (240 g) quick-cook oatmeal with 2 tbsp honey, 1 large banana, 4 oz (120 mL) juice
- 4-oz (115 g) bagel, 2 tbsp peanut butter, 2 tbsp jam, 12 oz (360 mL) juice
- 1 cup (190 g) rice (cooked) with honey, 2 tbsp peanut butter, 1 banana
- 1 cup (240 g) applesauce, 1-1/4 cup (35 g) rice crispy cereal, 2 tbsp peanut butter, 1 tbsp honey
- 1/2 cup (100 g) quinoa (cooked), 1/2 cup (115 g) sweet potato, 1 tsp olive oil, salt, pepper
- 1 sports bar (Lärabar or anything with low fat and little protein), 1 medium banana, 1 tbsp nut butter
- 4 oz (120 mL) juice, 1 small muffin, 1 banana, 1 tbsp nut butter
- 2 frozen waffles with 2 tbsp nut butter and maple syrup, 1 banana, 8-12 oz (240-360 mL) sports drink
- 2 pieces white toast with 1-2 tbsp nut butter, 1 banana, 8-12 oz (240-360 mL) sports drink

Tater Tots and Cheese With Furikake or Seeds

This recipe is good before a workout.
Servings: 2

Ingredients:
- 12 oz (345 g) Tater Tots (regular or sweet potato)
- 1 tbsp olive oil
- 1/4 tsp salt
- 2 oz (60 g) grated or shaved parmesan cheese
- 1 tbsp furikake or 2 tbsp mixed seeds (sunflower, hemp, chia, pumpkin, etc.)

Directions
1. Preheat oven to 400 °F (200 °C).
2. Remove Tater Tots from the package and empty onto a baking sheet.
3. Drizzle with oil and salt. Bake for 20 minutes or until crispy.
4. Portion into two servings.
5. Sprinkle with parmesan and furikake or seeds.

Tiramisu Overnight Oats

Try this hearty carbohydrate and caffeine energy boost at the start of a big training day.
Servings: 2

Ingredients

- 2 shots espresso (or instant coffee)
- 1 cup (80 g) rolled oats (dry)
- 2 tbsp chia seeds
- Pinch of kosher or sea salt
- 2/3 cup (160 mL) milk (cow's milk or alternative)
- 1/2 (115 g) cup yogurt
- 1 tbsp maple syrup
- 1 tsp vanilla extract or paste
- 1/4 cup (65 g) chocolate hazelnut butter (Justin's Chocolate Hazelnut and Almond Butter is a great choice)

Directions

1. Make the espresso and let it cool while you complete the next step.
2. In a bowl, add the rolled oats, chia seeds, and salt.
3. Add the maple syrup, vanilla extract, yogurt, milk, and half the espresso and stir well. Layer into jars.
4. Mix the chocolate hazelnut butter with the other half of the espresso and stir until combined.
5. Layer the hazelnut and espresso mixture evenly over the top of each jar.
6. Place in the fridge overnight.

Sample Three-Day Carb-Increase Menu for 150-Pound Athlete (Carb Needs: 477-818 g)

Day One

Breakfast: 3 waffles, 2 eggs, 1 banana

Snack 1: 1 cup (230 g) quick oats (cooked), fruit smoothie

Lunch: 1 cup (230 g) orzo salad with tofu, 1 medium roasted potato, 1/2 cup (120 g) applesauce

Snack 2: Handful of pretzel sticks, 1 pita, 3 tbsp hummus

Dinner: 2 oz (60 g) pasta with red sauce, 2 slices garlic bread

Snack 3: 8 oz (230 g) Greek yogurt with 1/2 cup (60 g) granola, 12 oz (360 mL) juice

Estimated Total Carbs: 545 g

Day Two

Breakfast: Fruit smoothie bowl topped with 1/2 cup (60 g) granola and chocolate chips

Snack 1: 1 Bobo's granola bar

Lunch: Turkey wrap, 2 cookies, 8 oz (240 mL) juice

Snack 2: Bowl of cereal with milk

Dinner: 2-3 slices pizza

Snack 3: 1 cup (230 g) sorbet, recovery shake

Estimated Total Carbs: 600 g

Day Three

Breakfast: 2 frozen waffles with nut butter and maple syrup, 1 banana

Snack 1: 16 oz (480 mL) sports drink, 5 dates

Lunch: 1.5-2 cups (300-400 g) pasta salad, 8 oz (240 mL) juice

Snack 2: 3 packets fruit snacks

Dinner: 1.5 cups (275 g) rice (cooked) with seasoned chicken

Snack 3: 2 cookies, 8 oz (240 mL) juice

Estimated Total Carbs: 625 g

Takeaways

- While fueling during workouts and races tends to be a focal area for many endurance athletes, maximizing your preworkout and prerace fueling offers an additional opportunity to capitalize on performance gains.

- Entering a workout or race underfueled or underhydrated can not only put you behind from the start, but in certain situations, the consequences can risk your health.

- Planning and testing preworkout and prerace fueling strategies can help you determine what likely will and will not work on race day and focus on what makes you feel the best overall.

- Regardless of what strategies you use, remember this saying: Never try anything new during race week.

9

NUTRITION NEEDS DURING YOUR WORKOUT OR RACE

It was the morning of the 2014 Chicago Marathon, and Matt Llano had just finished an intense training block. He was feeling good, ready to seek out a new PR. At every 5K interval, aid stations had bottles set out and ready to go. Instead of getting caught up in the commotion with other competitors, Matt decided to skip his bottles. At mile 21, his energy started to disappear, and the lead pack of runners faded away. He learned this lesson: Fuel often and fuel early.

You can never fully predict what will happen during a target event, but you can avoid mistakes *if* you take the time to optimize all the pieces of your individualized fueling plan, have backups and alternatives, test the plan, and understand how to listen to your body along the way.

The key is to choose the right fuel at the right time. Do a quick online search for the best sports nutrition products, and you'll get thousands of results. Unfortunately, with so many options, endurance athletes are left with a huge question about what they should be eating and drinking to fuel long training sessions and races. The short answer is that it depends. There are numerous factors at play: the duration, the intensity, the climate, your sweat rate, and your gut tolerance, to name a few. That's why you'll want to figure out your best, personalized plan well in advance of a goal event.

It started as an experiment. What would happen if the fluids and foods used to fuel athletes were made from scratch with certain principles in mind instead of using traditional sports fueling options that caused gastrointestinal issues? This is just what Dr. Allen Lim, founder of Skratch Labs hydration mix, learned when he began to make food and drinks that athletes used when training and racing—no gastrointestinal distress, less flavor fatigue, and better performance.

After many requests from athletes to get their hands on the hydration mixes, he was producing at home, he and his two friends Aaron Foster and Ian MacGregor decided to start making larger quantities of drink mix in a small at-home blender. Soon after, they moved on to food-safe paint buckets mixed in the paint shaker at their local hardware store. And from there, his experiments became so popular that he officially launched Skratch Labs in 2012 with the simple belief that no matter where you find yourself in life, you can always start from scratch.

Dr. Lim admits that in all the time he has spent in the endurance world working with athletes on their nutrition, the biggest mistake he sees athletes make is not having a plan for all possibilities in an event and not listening to their body when the plan needs to change. Which begs the important questions "What are the 'right' ways to fuel endurance events?", "Where do you even start?", and "How do you adjust when things go awry?"

Fuel for Your Activity

When planning for both your workouts and your races, there are several factors to keep in mind. It is of utmost importance to test out your fueling strategies during your training so you can see what works best for you and your body. Particularly when your workout or race will last longer than 60 minutes, pay close attention to the hydration, electrolytes, and overall energy needs for that day.

Hydration Losses

Fluids (from blood plasma, extracellular water, and intracellular water) play many important roles in the body. They help eliminate waste, balance electrolytes, carry nutrients, and regulate body temperature. When considering the impact that hydration has on exercise performance, we know that a decrease in blood plasma fluids can negatively affect exercise capacity and thermoregulation. Without enough fluids, blood flow to the skin decreases and heart rate increases (Shirreffs and Sawka 2011). Even small losses in overall body fluids can affect your ability to perform at higher intensities.

Sweat Composition

Each drop of sweat you lose contains positively and negatively charged ions, or electrolytes. Electrolytes help maintain proper fluid balance, support normal muscle contractions, and keep the body running smoothly overall. A lack of electrolytes during exercise can cause dysregulation of physiological processes such as heat tolerance, increase the chances of an energy crash while exercising, and lead to dizziness and disorientation. Sweat composition is highly individualized and contains predominantly sodium, chloride, magnesium, calcium, and phosphorus. Sodium is the electrolyte that is lost in the highest amounts in sweat, is found in the largest amounts in our intracellular space, and has the biggest impact on total body hydration status. When trying to determine fluid and electrolyte requirements during exercise, you only need to focus on sweat sodium concentration test results (Jeukendrup 2010). This is not to downplay the losses of other electrolytes, but those losses are much smaller and can typically be replaced in the diet. The exception to this may be during an ultra-endurance event, where magnesium, calcium, and potassium losses could create such a large hole that it affects performance. However, even then, many sports nutrition products and foods consumed will contain enough of these micronutrients to prevent having to have specific interworkout intake targets for them.

Sports Drink Recipes

If you want to make your own sports drink to replenish your carbohydrate and electrolyte stores, look no further than these homemade sports drinks.

Pineapple Lime Hydrator

Ingredients
- 2 cups (480 mL) water
- 1 cup (240 mL) pineapple juice
- 1 tbsp lime juice
- 1/8 tsp salt

Directions
1. Mix all ingredients together in a pitcher.
2. Drink up!

Maple Quencher

Ingredients
- 3-3/4 cup (900 mL) cold water
- 1/4 cup (85 g) pure maple syrup
- 1/4 tsp salt

Directions
1. Mix all ingredients together in a pitcher.
2. Drink up!

Mint Grape Refresher

Ingredients

- 2 cups (480 mL) brewed mint tea, cooled
- 1 cup (240 mL) 100% grape juice
- 1 tbsp lemon juice
- 1/8 tsp salt

Directions

1. Mix all ingredients together in a pitcher.
2. Drink up!

Energy Intake

Think of calories as the energy or gas to fuel your system. Your body has a limited amount of stored carbohydrate in its muscles and liver (only 1,800 to 2,000 calories' worth, depending on body frame size and diet). Once these are emptied, the body relies on fat and protein (muscle breakdown) to fuel itself, which is a slower process, causing you to have less energy and increasing your risk of an energy crash or "bonk" during exercise. To keep this from happening, consume at least 30 grams of carbohydrate per hour during exercise—but this can be increased to up to 90 grams per hour before the gastrointestinal system becomes more taxed. Keep in mind that if you are taking in higher amounts of carbohydrate per hour, varying the sugar types (glucose and fructose) is recommended due to the limited number of individual transporters (Bergström et al. 1967).

An average endurance athlete can easily expend 600 to 1,000 calories per hour during training and racing. A good target is to replace around 30 to 40 percent of those calories, which means consuming 180 to 400 calories per hour. Remember that calories can come from a variety of sources such as hydration mixes, gels, chews, food blends, and whole foods. You must be strategic about logistics, palatability, and portability of calorie choices depending on your target race.

Options for Fueling

Experiment with different types of fuels to have with you during your workout or race. For longer endurance events, is important to have variety so you don't experience palate fatigue.

- *Sports gels:* Conveniently packaged and easy to carry, these carbohydrate sources allow endurance athletes to fuel themselves quickly while training and racing. Sports gels are usually absorbed quickly and prevent blood sugar from dropping too much. Pay attention to the sugar types used in different gels, and be careful with additives such as vitamins, minerals, and caffeine to avoid gastrointestinal distress.

• *Energy chews:* Similar to sports gels but reminiscent of gummy candy, chews are specifically designed to be convenient blocks of chewable energy. They are perfect for the athlete who doesn't like the texture of gels or wants something solid to chew on for energy intake.

• *Hydration mixes:* For the endurance athlete who wants to drink their calories, these mixes are specially formulated as a vehicle for calories, carbohydrates, and electrolytes. They are perfect for the endurance athlete who can't seem to eat gels, chews, or solid foods as much during training and racing.

Potatoes provide a high amount of carbohydrates per portion.

loops7/Getty Images

• *Whole-food sources:* Exactly as described, whole-food options are foods that endurance athletes can use during exercise to fuel their activities. These are a good choice for distances longer than a marathon and allow athletes to mix up their fuel sources, so they don't end up with stomach distress. As a reminder, blood is diverted away from the gut during exercise, so the higher your intensity, the less you will digest. Use caution when eating whole foods during high-intensity exercise. See table 9.1 for whole-food options.

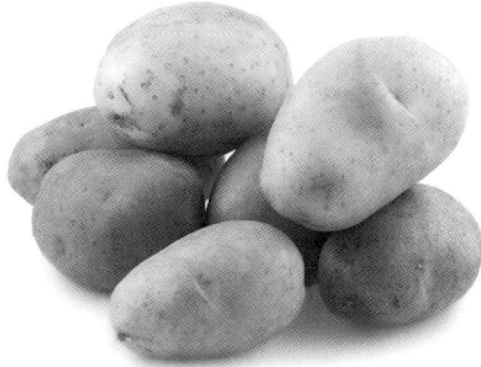

TABLE 9.1   Whole-Food Options for Fueling

Food option and serving size	Calories	Carbo-hydrate	Protein	Fat	Sodium
Fig cookies (2)	110	22 g	1 g	2 g	95 mg
PB&J sandwich (1)	210	28 g	6 g	9 g	220 mg
Medjool dates (2)	133	36 g	1 g	0 g	0 mg
Boiled baby red potatoes with salt (2)	210	54 g	6 g	0 g	220 mg
Pierogi (3)	270	44 g	5 g	6 g	550 mg
Banana bread (1 piece)	247	39 g	2 g	9 g	110 mg
Nut butter packet (1)	190	8 g	7 g	16 g	130 mg
Chocolate chip cookie (1)	148	20 g	0.6 g	7.4 g	91 mg
Salted soft pretzel bites (4)	117	24 g	3 g	1 g	712 mg
Tortilla rollup with 2 tbsp jam (1)	251	53 g	4 g	3 g	434 mg
Salted plantain chips (20)	140	20 g	1 g	7 g	75 mg
Bao bun (1)	114	22 g	3 g	2 g	2 mg
Pancakes (2 small)	198	27 g	6 g	8 g	612 mg
Oatmeal cream pie (1)	170	26 g	1 g	7 g	190 mg
Rice Krispies Treats (1)	116	21 g	0 g	3 g	129 mg
Oreos (3)	161	25 g	2 g	7 g	140 mg

(continued)

TABLE 9.1   *(continued)*

Food option and serving size	Calories	Carbo-hydrate	Protein	Fat	Sodium
Belgian Liège waffles (1)	230	30 g	5 g	10 g	200 mg
Salted rice balls (2)	126	16 g	2 g	8 g	200 mg
Pop-Tarts (1)	200	38 g	2 g	5 g	170 mg

Whole-Food Recipes for Workout Fueling by Kelly Newlon of Real Athlete Diets (RAD) in Boulder, Colorado

Both these recipes are fun and unexpected and have great texture and flavor. They are easy and can be made in batches and frozen. Because of their more complex nutrition profiles (carbohydrates, proteins, and fats), they are better fueling options for ultra-endurance events.

Sticky Rice Spring Rolls

Makes approximately 6 spring rolls.

Ingredients

- 1 cup (230 g) glutinous rice (short grain, like sushi rice) (cooked)
- 1/2 cup (130 g) peanut butter
- 2 tbsp tamari soy
- 2 tbsp honey
- 1 tbsp water
- 1 tsp sesame seeds
- 1 tbsp rice vinegar
- 1/2 cup (40 g) chopped or shredded red cabbage
- 1/4 cup (28 g) chopped or shredded carrots
- 1/4 cup (30 g) chopped cucumber
- 1/2 cup (115 g) chopped protein (tofu, chicken, pork, shrimp, etc.)
- Rice paper

Directions

1. Cook rice and set aside to cool.
2. Mix peanut butter, tamari, honey, water, sesame seeds, and rice vinegar until smooth.
3. Roughly chop vegetables and protein.
4. Add sauce, vegetables, and protein to rice and mix until just combined, being careful not to overwork the rice.
5. Build spring rolls and enjoy before, during, or after activity.

Professional Chef/Sports Nutrition.

Brown Rice Spanakopita

Ingredients

- 1 cup (240 mL) olive or avocado oil for brushing and building spanakopita
- 1 lb (460 g) phyllo dough, thawed (usually 1 box)
- 1 tsp kosher or sea salt
- 1/4 tsp ground black pepper
- 4 oz (125 g) feta, goat, or plant-based alternative cheese
- 2 cups (380 g) cooked brown rice
- 1/2 avocado, gently smashed
- 1 tsp lemon juice
- 1 cup (180 g) spinach (cooked, drained, chopped, and cooled)
- 1 egg, beaten (or 3 tbsp Just Egg)

Directions

1. Preheat oven to 375 °F (190 °C).
2. Set oil and phyllo dough aside.
3. Add all other ingredients to a large bowl and mix until evenly combined.
4. Take the phyllo dough out of the package and unroll it onto a flat surface. Keep the dough covered with plastic wrap or a damp towel when you're not working with it.
5. Lay out one sheet of dough with the long end facing you. Brush oil all over the dough.
6. Add a second layer of dough on top of the first, then brush the second layer with oil.
7. Cut the dough vertically into strips 3 in. (9 cm) wide.
8. Place 1-1/2 tsp of filling on one end of a dough strip. Fold one corner of the dough over the filling to make a triangle.
9. Fold the strip of dough over itself the same way you would fold a flag until you reach the end.
10. Brush a little oil over the top and place the triangle on a prepared baking sheet.
11. Repeat the process with the remaining dough and filling.
12. Arrange the triangles 1-1/2 in. (4.5 cm) apart on baking sheets. Bake one sheet at a time for 18-20 minutes or until golden brown.

These can be made ahead of time and frozen until you want to bake them or baked and kept in the freezer for up to one month. They are great to add to a salad, snack on at home, or wrap individually in foil to take on the trail.

Professional Chef/Sports Nutrition.

Carrying It All

A big challenge that many endurance athletes face once they choose their race fueling options is how to carry it all. Here are some of the tools I've found most helpful for endurance athletes:

- *Race belt:* Though not incredibly spacious, these convenient, lightweight belts allow you to squeeze in a soft flask and go hands-free, with additional room for some sports nutrition products.

- *Hydration pack:* More spacious, these backpacks can hold a lot of fluid volume as well as nutrition. Most packs let you carry a bladder of fluid on your back and bottles on the front. They're great for long or multiday endurance adventures.

- *Handheld water bottle:* Great for shorter bouts of exercise, these bottles are a quick way to transport fluids (and they may or may not have a pocket to carry nutrition).

- *Filter bottle:* Think of these bottles as a way to ensure you can get in fluids no matter where you are training. With a unique filter cap, they allow you to scoop water from lakes, streams, and even puddles. They are a great option for the backcountry or situations where you don't want to carry a lot of fluids.

- *Bike frame hydration reservoir:* Perfect for cyclists who want to carry more on their bike for longer adventures and training sessions, these reservoirs are fitted to the bike and can carry large amounts of fluids.

Putting It All Together

Once you have figured out all the components of your fueling plan and how you will carry everything, you must get the timing right. Regular intake of calories, fluids, and electrolytes is an important part of fueling success. Some endurance athletes get caught up in the energy of racing or experience a lack of appetite or thirst, which doesn't make it easy to get it all in.

You may decide to take in fuel regularly in 10-, 20-, or 30-minute intervals, but no matter what, it is important to have a pattern that works for you and that you will remember. Setting a watch alarm as a reminder when you practice your fueling plan can help you accomplish your goal of getting all your fuel in on time, so you don't get behind.

Because of the fickle nature of your gastrointestinal system and the complicated task of combining all the pieces of your fueling plan, it is recommended that you begin testing all fueling plan components two to three months before your target race so you can make the necessary adjustments ahead of time. Lay out your components on a detailed fueling plan chart that breaks down your hourly nutrition analysis to visualize your options, portions, and pattern of intake.

Table 9.2 can be a useful tool for planning what you will consume throughout your activity. There are multiple sections of the chart with similar labels because you will need to consider the hypothetical hours of your event and the fuel sources you are choosing to put together.

Here are some tips for using this chart:

1. For longer races, consider mixing up fuel sources to include savory and sweet options.

2. Consider mixing up your sports nutrition product flavors and textures. Providing different options can help prevent palate fatigue from occurring.

3. For longer races (over three hours), include three to five whole-food options in your plan. Building in more food options than this can cause confusion and make it harder to execute the plan.

4. It can be helpful to include hydration mixes with and without calories in case you end up in a situation where you don't want to consume something sweet.

5. Consider your portions. Make sure you include the food portion size you are consuming to get in the right nutrition needed each hour.

6. For triathlons, you may want to build in fueling options to have in the transition area between the swim and bike and the bike and run.

7. Include possible aid station options and the portions you will need. This can help in two instances: if you don't want to carry as much with you or if you want to pivot and use fuel from the course instead of what you brought.

Fueling Plan Testing Tips

Allow yourself enough time to test your fueling plan and ensure all the possible hourly options will work logistically and with your stomach.

- Only test one hourly combination at a time when starting out. For instance, if you are doing a three-hour run, only use the products from one of the hours on your chart to fuel the entire run. This allows you to troubleshoot possible problem areas.

- Once all the hours have been tested individually, you can test different hours together to ensure the products will work congruently in your fueling plan.

TABLE 9.2   Fueling Plan Chart

During long race or workout	Hydration options	Gels or chews	Food option	Food option	Totals	Targets
Calories						
Carbohydrate						
Sodium						
Protein						
Fat						
Calories						
Carbohydrate						
Sodium						
Protein						
Fat						
Calories						
Carbohydrate						
Sodium						
Protein						
Fat						
Calories						
Carbohydrate						
Sodium						
Protein						
Fat						

From K. Van Horn, *Practical Fueling for Endurance Athletes: Your Nutrition Guide for Optimal Performance*, (Champaign, IL: Human Kinetics, 2026).

Whole-Food Blend Recipes for Fueling

If you are looking for a good alternative to sports gels that you can make at home, these whole-food blends provide the carbohydrates you need for fueling. Put all food blends in a reusable flask to take them during your training sessions.

Banana Date Food Blend

Servings: 3

Ingredients
- 1 medium banana
- 3 dates
- 3/4 cup (180 mL) water
- Pinch of salt

Directions
1. Soak dates in water for 30 minutes.
2. Puree banana, dates, and soaking liquid until smooth.
3. Add a pinch of salt.
4. Add water, 1 tbsp at a time, if too thick.
5. Store up to three days in the fridge.

Nutrition Facts (Per Serving)

Calories: 101

Carbs: 27 g

Sodium: 52 mg

Potassium: 308 mg

Banana Sweet Potato Food Blend

Servings: 2

Ingredients
- 1/2 cup (115 g) roasted or steamed sweet potato (peeled)
- 1 medium banana
- 1/4 tsp salt
- 1/2 cup (120 mL) water, plus additional water

Directions
1. Puree sweet potato, banana, salt, and 1/2 cup (120 mL) water until smooth.
2. Add more water, 1 tbsp at a time, to achieve desired texture.
3. Store up to three days in the fridge.

Nutrition Facts (Per Serving)

Calories: 109

Carbs: 27 g

Sodium: 311 mg

Potassium: 514 mg

Maple Apple Cinnamon

Servings: 2

Ingredients

- 1 cup (240 g) unsweetened applesauce
- 2 tbsp maple syrup
- 1/2 cup (120 mL) water, plus additional water
- Pinch of salt

Directions

1. Puree applesauce, maple syrup, 1/2 cup (120 mL) water, and salt.
2. Add more water, 1 tbsp at a time, to achieve desired texture.
3. Store up to three days in the fridge.

Nutrition Facts (Per Serving)

Calories: 102

Carbs: 27 g

Sodium: 82 mg

Potassium: 132 mg

Peanut Butter Sweet Potato Food Blend

Servings: 2

Ingredients

- 1/2 cup (115 g) roasted or steamed sweet potato (peeled)
- 1 tbsp peanut butter
- Dash of salt
- 1/2 cup (120 mL) water, plus additional water

Directions

1. Puree sweet potato, peanut butter, salt, and 1/2 cup (120 mL) water until smooth.
2. Add more water, 1 tbsp at a time, to achieve desired texture.
3. Store up to three days in the fridge.

Nutrition Facts (Per Serving)

Calories: 105

Carbs: 15 g

Sodium: 135 mg

Potassium: 348 mg

Piña Colada Food Blend

Servings: 2

Ingredients

- 1 banana
- 1/2 cup (125 g) frozen or fresh pineapple
- 2 tbsp shredded coconut
- 1/2 cup (120 mL) coconut water
- 1/4 tsp salt

Directions

1. Puree banana, pineapple, shredded coconut, coconut water, and salt until smooth.
2. Add water, 1 tbsp at a time, to achieve desired texture.
3. Store up to three days in the fridge.

Nutrition Facts (Per Serving)

Calories: 102

Carbs: 27 g

Sodium: 314 mg

Potassium: 66 mg

Race-Day Nutrition

One of the greatest performance-enhancing strategies that endurance athletes can implement on race day is choosing to fuel appropriately with the correct fluid amounts, electrolytes, and calorie options. You need to factor in sport-specific considerations for your logistical planning and implementation to succeed. For instance, an ultramarathoner naively thinking that they can use only gels for the entire event can lead to problematic palate fatigue and nausea later in the race. Conversely, solid food options during a road marathon may be difficult for the body to process and could lead to stomach cramping and distress.

Taking the time to practice the fueling options you have organized for your race-day plan is crucial for figuring out whether your strategies and backup strategies will carry you through on the big day. Use the following sport-specific recommendations to guide your fueling plan for race day and adapt as needed.

Fueling for Races Shorter Than One Hour (5K and 10K Distances)

Planning for shorter distance events of less than an hour requires much less time and effort than their longer distance counterparts. While some athletes might feel better if they fuel during these distances, heavy fueling strategies are optional. A robust prerace fueling plan may benefit you more than a during-the-race strategy here, but keep in mind that all athletes respond uniquely and require different amounts to feel their best.

- Calorie intake is optional, but some athletes may feel better consuming carbohydrates during these races. If you plan on taking in some calories during the race, be sure to carry them with you because there may not be any on-course nutrition.

- Hydration may be helpful during shorter events, especially if it is hot or you have high fluid loss rates. You could carry a handheld water bottle, or if there will be any water stations on the course, you can get fluids there. Be sure to practice drinking from aid station cups ahead of time, or you will end up pouring it all over yourself. Remember, pinch the top, pour it in your mouth, and go!

- Sports drinks are also optional during shorter events, but even just rinsing your mouth with a sports drink can provide a boost of energy midrace.

- For shorter events, glycogen stores are less likely to empty, so carbohydrate consumption can range from 30 to 60 grams per hour.

Fueling for Longer Distance Events (Marathons, 42Ks, and Endurance Cycling Races)

Whether you are training to finish your 1st or 50th marathon, the distance is an entirely different thing than shorter distance events like the 5K, 10K, or even half-marathon. Whatever your goals or reasons for going the distance, a well-planned fueling and hydration strategy can determine whether you hit the dreaded wall at mile 20 of your race, forcing you to walk to the finish line, or not. Regardless of your speed, you must figure out how to time your hydration and calorie consumption along the racecourse. Many marathoners are concerned about the impact of carrying fuel and opt to use racecourse options instead to save weight and time.

Whatever you decide to do, remember that you absolutely need to be testing race-day nutrition products throughout your long training runs. Research the race ahead of time and email the organizers to ask what products will be used on the racecourse if you plan on using them. Here's a word of caution, though: If you are planning on using nutrition products provided by the race, expect that things such as hydration mixes may not be mixed to your desired or practiced concentration. This could backfire and lead to gastrointestinal distress or even bonking (if weakly prepared). If you choose to carry your own products, it is important to figure out how you will carry everything.

Race conditions can also vary on race day, so practicing in various weather conditions is important, too, if possible. Work on an intentional carbohydrate intake strategy ahead of time to get an invaluable performance enhancement.

Guidelines for Fluid, Calorie, and Electrolyte Consumption

The longer endurance events get, the more important an intentional strategy becomes. Gaps in hydration, electrolytes, and calorie consumption can lead to bigger effects over the course of a three-hour period than during a 5K. Aim for the following targets to optimize your fueling plan.

Fluids

- *Have a plan:* Plan and practice your fluid intake strategy. You want to take in small amounts of fluid regularly, not one big gulp all at once. Typical intake patterns range from 3 to 4 ounces every 10 minutes to 6 to 8 ounces every 15 minutes.

- *Know your fluid loss rate:* Know your fluid loss rate ahead of the race. If the race is hotter, more humid, or at a high altitude, you may need to adjust accordingly. You should not gain weight during exercise. If you do, it could indicate that

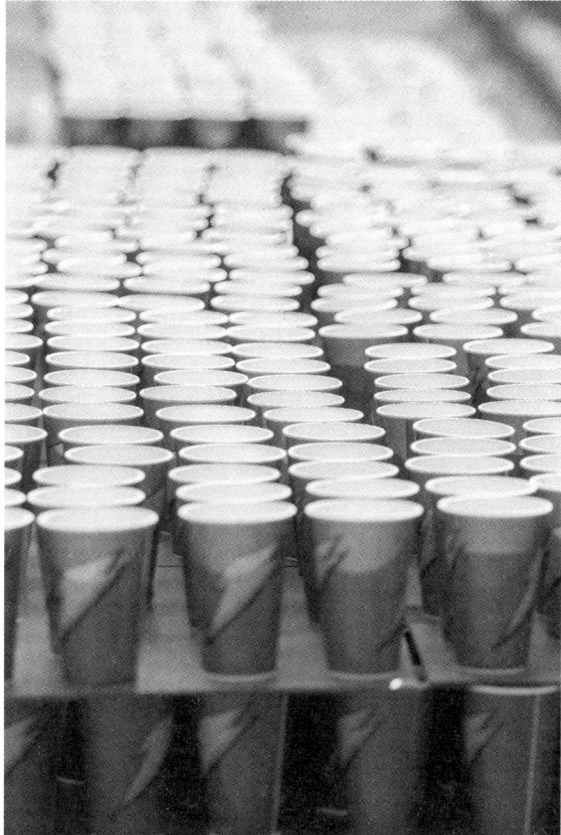

If you do not carry your own fluids, know how far apart the aid stations appear on the course and plan for your target fluid consumption at the different stops.

you are consuming too much fluid every hour and are at risk of hyponatremia.

- *Scope out the aid stations ahead of time:* Be sure you know what fluid and calorie options will be served at the event aid stations. Knowing how far apart the aid stations will be can help you plan your fluid consumption.
- *Decide if you will carry your own fluids:* Determine beforehand whether you will carry your own fluids or get some from the course. Be aware that if you are planning on using the hydration mix on the course, it may not be mixed to the proper concentration, which could increase the risk of stomach distress.

Fuel Sources

- Exogenous carbohydrate consumption is recommended during endurance exercise lasting longer than 90 minutes to help offset glycogen depletion.
- For races you expect to finish in three hours or less, aim for 30 to 60 grams of carbohydrate per hour. For races longer than three hours, you should take in 60 to 90 grams of carbohydrate per hour.
- Aim to get your carbohydrates from varied sources (glucose and fructose) if possible due to the limited capacity of glucose and fructose transporters in the small intestine.
- Carbohydrates for this distance can come from gels, chews, candy, soda, and hydration mixes; whole-food sources in a marathon could be harder to digest and are not recommended.
- Begin consuming carbohydrates early and often for performance benefits. Different products contain different amounts of carbohydrate, so be aware of this and take in products at regular intervals to meet your calorie needs every hour.

Electrolytes

- Sodium and electrolyte intake during exercise may benefit endurance athletes who are racing in particularly hot, humid, or high-altitude conditions and have high sweat sodium losses.
- There are not consistent recommendations for sodium intake during marathon-distance events, but you want to ensure your sodium intake matches your fluid replenishment rates. If you consume too much sodium, it could lead to nausea and vomiting.
- Your body may absorb fluids best and use your carbohydrate intake more effectively if you have some sodium with your fluids. If you can't get a sweat sodium test done, try to consume a minimum of 250 milligrams of sodium every hour.
- If you're using electrolyte capsules, be careful so you don't overwhelm your system. Try not to consume too many at one time, and ensure you take them with fluid.

Fueling for Sport-Specific Long-Course Endurance Events

When you're looking to optimize performance at marathon-distance events, take into account any sport-specific considerations. Logistical mistakes can derail all your efforts to successfully complete these types of events, which include marathons, cycling endurance races, and long-course triathlons.

Marathon

- It is important for marathon runners to be keenly aware of the number of water or aid stations on the course. If you are not planning on carrying your own fluids, you will need to plan your stops appropriately. It can be helpful to practice drinking out of race cups (pinch the top) in your training, so you don't dump the fluids all over your face. Be sure to bring enough of your sports nutrition products with you. If you plan on using sports gels on the course, be sure to check whether all the aid stations will have them or only some. If you are bringing your own gels, bring a few extra just in case the race takes you a little longer than you anticipated.

- Elite runners who have the privilege of having their own fluid tables must be sure that their bottles are decorated and distinct from the others. Bright, easily recognizable colors can help set them apart in a sea of other bottles.

- If you are participating in a trail race, consider wearing a hydration pack so you can carry a lot of fluids and fuel sources in case the aid stations are spread out. If the aid stations are spread thin, be sure to set fueling reminders on your watch so you don't forget to fuel.

Cycling

- Be sure to know your fluid losses so you can predict how much fluid you need to carry and aim to consume every hour. Logistically speaking, road cyclists going longer distances may need to install water reservoirs on their bikes.

- Liquid calories in the form of hydration mixes can be a convenient way to get in calories and electrolytes while on a bike. However, for events lasting longer than two to three hours, it's a good idea to take in more solid food.

- You will likely be carrying much of your own fuel in your jersey pockets unless there is an option to get aid at feed zone areas along the course.

- A power meter is a device mounted on a bike that measures the power produced by the cyclist. This is a helpful tool to determine hourly energy expenditure and, consequently, hourly target calorie intake. Aim to take in 40 to 50 percent of your energy burned every hour.

- Be smart about the timing of your fuel intake. Don't take in too much at the bottom of a hill you're about to climb.

Long-Course Triathlon (Ironman 70.3 and Ironman)
Because of the multisport nature of these longer triathlon events, it can take a bit more planning and logistics to develop a fueling strategy that will work on race day. Unlike with shorter races or single-sport events, you may need to vary your fuel choices, and the logistical variables of carrying your fuel can determine the race outcome.

Some of the main nutrition challenges for long-course triathlons stem from the following:

- Dehydration from not taking in enough fluids throughout the race
- Gastrointestinal distress from swallowing too much water during the swim or making wrong fueling choices
- Bonking, or having low energy, from running out of fuel, which makes you slow down or stop
- Failure to adjust the fueling plan to the current weather and race terrain

Pay close attention to the following details, which are required for a fueling plan for these multisport races.

Calorie Intake

Calorie intake during long-course triathlon events should equate to roughly 30 to 50 percent of your energy expenditure. While you can use a power meter on your bike to figure out your specific target range, this typically equates to between 200 and 400 calories per hour for most triathletes. Remember, duration, terrain, and intensity affect your energy burned every hour—hence the importance of adapting your fueling plan to the race. Carbohydrates should still be the predominant calorie source, but you may be able to tolerate a little protein and fat during the bike portion of your race.

Triathlon Nutrition for the Swimming Portion

In general, be prepared for the swim to be a bit chaotic. Many athletes find that they swallow excessive amounts of water, which can make them feel sick when they make it to the transition. In extreme cases, some athletes feel seasick in open-water swims. To combat these problems, practice breathing techniques ahead of time and be prepared with something to quell your stomach, such as ginger chews or peppermints.

Triathlon Nutrition for the Cycling Portion

The cycling portion of a triathlon is the longest portion of the race. Because of the reduced gastrointestinal jostling during this portion of the race, it can be beneficial to try to take in more calories and solid foods than you will during the run. Some athletes feel better mixing up their fueling plan and using potatoes, cookies, or bars instead of the traditional gels or chews. If you tend to feel sick on the run, you may feel better if you use all-liquid nutrition toward the end of the cycling portion (30 to 60 minutes remaining) before you transition to the run. You may be able to tolerate more carbohydrate per hour on the bike than on the run because of the jostling during the run. Plan your nutrition accordingly. Be sure to know your fluid loss rate ahead of time so you can anticipate hydration requirements during the cycling. If you have high fluid replenishment requirements, you need to make sure you have the carrying capacity, maybe mounting an extra bottle cage to your bike.

Triathlon Nutrition for the Running Portion

The running portion of a triathlon is typically where the most stomach issues occur because of the stressful transition from cycle to running. Remember that solid foods you may have used on the bike likely will not work well on the run. A strategy that works well is setting up your fueling plan to anticipate slightly lower calorie intake per hour during the run. Be sure to continue consuming calories and fluids during this portion, or you can end up bonking or crawling to the finish line. If you truly cannot consume your planned sports nutrition products, try

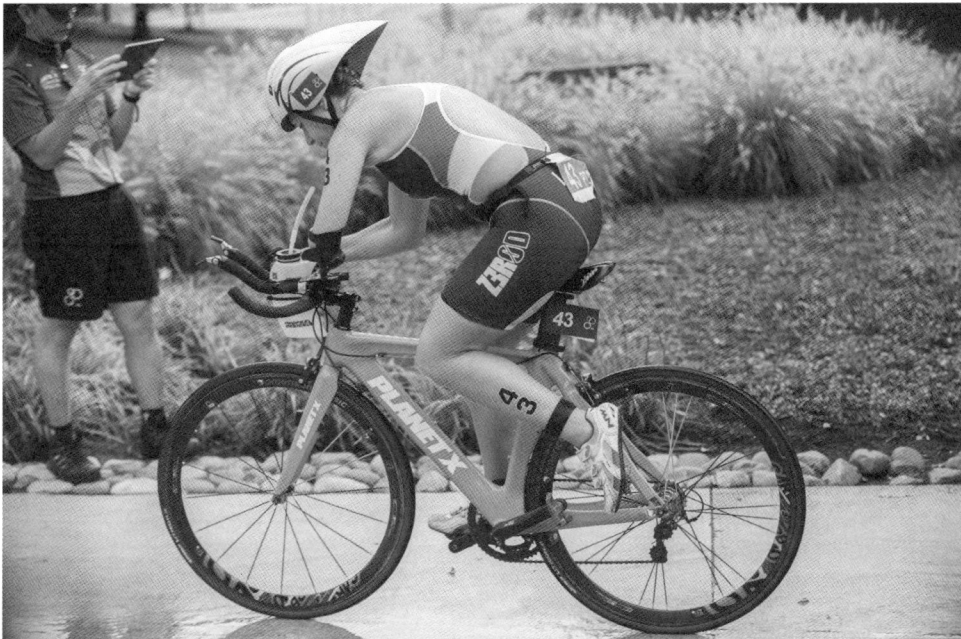

Plan to mount an extra bottle cage to your bike for hydration during the cycling portion of the race if you have high fluid replenishment requirements.

letting a piece of hard candy sit in your mouth to see if your stomach will calm down.

What About Transitions?

For some endurance athletes, transitions are a time when they get in a little extra nutrition and calm down their breathing and heart rate before starting the next portion of the race. You might consider consuming some sort of sports nutrition product during this time, especially in the first transition after the swim, since you haven't had any intake for a while. Make sure to set up your transition area ahead of time and organize any nutrition products or hydration you want to use. It can be helpful to have a bottle filled with water or hydration mix so you can sip it while you transition. Pay attention to your intake during transitions to ensure you aren't taking in too much nutrition as you move into the cycling or running portions of your race.

Table 9.3 can be helpful for long-course triathletes to fill out ahead of time to practice their fueling options for each portion of the race (including transitions). The time estimates can help you predict how much fuel you will need to get enough calories per hour.

TABLE 9.3 Long-Course Triathlon Fueling Chart

	Time	Product	Total calories	Total carbs	Total sodium
Swim		None	None	None	None
Transition 1					
Cycling					
Transition 2					
Run					
Total time					
Total calories/hour					
Total carbs/hour					
Cycling carbs/hour					
Run carbs/hour					
Total sodium/hour					

From K. Van Horn, *Practical Fueling for Endurance Athletes: Your Nutrition Guide for Optimal Performance,* (Champaign, IL: Human Kinetics, 2026).

Ultramarathon Fueling

In the 2017 Tunnel Hill 100-Miler, Camille Herron broke the female world record for the 100-mile distance by over an hour. It was during this race that she switched from taking in 30 to 60 grams of carbohydrate per hour to taking in 60 to 90 grams of carbohydrate per hour, pushing her *calorie* limits over time. She credits the high-carb Maurten Drink Mix 320 for part of her success, citing that it was like "rocket fuel" powering her to take the record (athlete interview). Since then, she has pushed the boundaries of her fueling, ensuring that in all her ultra events, she takes in more calories rather than less.

For the purposes of this book, we will define ultradistance racing as anything longer than a marathon, which includes single-stage 50Ks, 50-milers, 100Ks, 100-milers, and beyond. These events require a wholly unique nutrition strategy, and it is important to remember that what worked for a marathon likely will not work for an ultramarathon event. Eating for ultradistance events is often referred to as a "walking picnic" because your pace tends to be slower and you are consuming nutrition throughout the entire day, not just for a few hours. Failing to prepare and practice a fueling plan specific to ultradistance events could be costly and often leads to more DNFs.

When you start the race, remember that you will be out there for a *long time*. This means that you are not going to be able to replace everything you are burning during the race. The goal, however, is to minimize calorie deficits while racing.

Keep in mind that you will be racing at a lower percentage of your $\dot{V}O_2$max than during marathon distance and shorter. This can allow you to take in more fuel every hour than you may be used to during shorter races. In a study done on 16 Western States Endurance Run (100 miles) finishers and nonfinishers, those who consumed less than 200 calories per hour were less likely to finish than those who did (Tiller et al. 2019). Recommended intake ranges from 150 to 400 calories per hour, depending on the event duration; however, prolonged intake (for the entire race) of less than 200 calories per hour is not recommended because it can increase the risk of nausea and vomiting.

• Recommended carbohydrate intake ranges from 30 to 90 grams per hour. Keep in mind that 90 grams of carbohydrate per hour may be difficult to maintain during ultradistance events and that using both carbohydrate and fat in your fueling plan may help you avoid gastrointestinal distress. If you are consuming more than 60 grams of carbohydrate per hour, it is important to evaluate your fueling plan and ensure you are using multiple transportable types of carbohydrate (glucose and fructose) to take advantage of the limited carbohydrate transporters. While some elite endurance athletes might be pushing the limits of carbohydrate intake during exercise (consuming up to 120-140g of carbohydrates per hour), this strategy is not recommended for most endurance athletes at this time due to the increased risk of gastrointestinal distress.

• Fats can be a viable option during ultra-endurance events to carry more calorie-dense foods without as much bulk and weight.

• Although protein plays a secondary role in energy production, during ultra-endurance events, it may be important for mitigating muscle protein breakdown, though this has not been confirmed in current research studies. If you are aiming to get some protein during races, consume smaller amounts (8 to 10 grams per hour) so you do not overwhelm your digestive system.

Consider the palatability of the foods you plan to consume during an ultra-endurance event. Your tastes and food preferences will likely change throughout the course of an ultradistance event. Studies show that as a race progresses, athletes crave fattier and saltier foods. The mechanism for this is unknown, but it is speculated that it is due to a chemical imbalance in the body or taste fatigue (Glace, Murphy, and McHugh 2002).

Athletes must consider the role aid stations will play in their fueling plan. Many aid stations at ultra-endurance events have a full-on food buffet, so it can be helpful to know ahead of time what will be offered so you can practice with some of the options in your own training. If the information is not readily available online, email the race director(s) to ask. It can also help to figure out the calorie content of aid station options beforehand to ensure you will get enough nutrition from what you grab (e.g., 2 pretzel twists have much fewer calories that 20 twists). Use caution with aid station options that are fried, have high protein, or contain dairy because these may lead to an upset stomach.

Hydration strategies for ultra-endurance events need to be highly individualized. Regular fluid loss testing is recommended. Keep in mind that fluid requirements can change; consider the race-day weather conditions, time of day or night, and altitude so you can plan your fluid intake pattern appropriately. Find out where the water stations will be located on the course, so you know how much fluid you need to carry between aid stations. To reduce the risk of hyponatremia during ultra-endurance racing, it is important to consume some electrolytes, particularly sodium, every hour during the event. In general, you should consume 300 to 600 milligrams of sodium every hour, but individual sweat sodium concentrations vary greatly. Consider doing sweat sodium concentration testing to figure out a personalized sodium intake pattern that works best for you.

Gastrointestinal distress in ultra-endurance racing is common, with an estimated 30 to 50 percent of ultra-endurance athletes experiencing some form of nausea, vomiting, diarrhea, or cramping during their race (de Oliveira, Burini, and Jeukendrup 2014). Navigating gastrointestinal distress in the middle of an ultra event can be tricky. You may need your crew members (family, friends, and loved ones) to help you because you may not have much mental clarity halfway through an ultra. For instance, if you're nauseated, you may want to continue taking in calories to see if it helps. It is important to keep a slow drip of calories coming into the system. Hydration mixes, hard candies, and chews can help accomplish this. Switching to a savory fueling option or plain water may also help if you are struggling with stomach distress. Carrying and taking stomach-neutralizing medications such as Pepto-Bismol or Tums can quell nausea to some extent, but it will not completely solve the issue.

You should carefully plan your caffeine consumption during any ultra-endurance race. Factor in your individual caffeine response because too much caffeine can cause gastrointestinal distress. If you are planning on consuming caffeine, it is advisable to do it during the night, when your circadian rhythm may be disrupted. If you're taking single doses of caffeine, you should be able to tolerate three to six milligrams per kilogram of body weight per hour, but more is not necessarily better. If you're taking multiple doses in a row, it is best to be more conservative and only take in one to two milligrams per kilogram of body weight every hour.

Other tips for ultramarathons include the following:

- Be prepared for the unknown on race day. Bringing a toothbrush and toothpaste to use midrace can help refresh the mouth and revive you during a low moment.

- Sucking on sour or spicy candies can recharge the palate or encourage saliva production if you are experiencing dry mouth.

- Lay out your fueling plan ahead of time to it easier for you and your crew to stay on track with what you need at aid stations.

- Pack your calorie bags before race day. This will allow you to keep track of your hourly intake and make it easier for your crew (if allowed) to give you what you need.

- Know your body and what you can tolerate during training and racing. A bean burrito may work for one athlete but go terribly for another.

- Have alternative fluid options for yourself. Don't carry only hydration mix and hope it will carry you through the entire event. Change it up with plain water, decarbonated cola, ginger ale, or sparkling water.

- When you leave an aid station, remember that if you just ate a plate of food, you likely do not need something else right away.

Ultramarathon Race-Day Fueling Tips From Camille

1. *Carry enough fluids and know what you need to replace:* We know it's possible to take in 60 to 90 grams of carbohydrate (glucose and fructose) per hour in whatever form works for you. It takes a lot of water to continue maximizing carbohydrate intake over time and keep the concentration in the gut diluted. It's important to experiment with quantities and your tolerance levels during long-distance training prior to the event. I personally try to stay on the low end of what's recommended (60 to 75 grams per hour) and only take in more if I feel like I need more.

2. *Space out your fuel:* I sip a sports drink every 10 to 15 minutes and set my watch to alert me to take a gel with water every 30 minutes. As the distance gets longer, you may need to consider adding whole-food sources or some protein. We always have food alternatives (such as fruit, potatoes, sports drinks or Maurten, soda, ginger beer, beer, sparkling mineral water, or sweet iced tea) or work with what's available at aid stations.

3. *Having treats to perk you up is always nice:* Whatever floats your boat! I've sometimes had tacos, burritos, pizza, or whatever sounds good at aid stations.

4. *Know how to fuel in the heat:* If the race is hot, I personally prefer to take in mainly liquids and gels. I tend to get nauseated when I eat solids in the heat. Ice-cold ginger beer or real beer are nice during hot races. I use insulated flasks to keep fluids cold.

5. *Carry your own goody bag and be cautious with caffeine use:* I like to carry NoDoz caffeine, Tums, and Hammer Endurolytes in case I run into issues on the course. I am sensitive to caffeine, so I usually only take half a NoDoz pill approximately one hour before the race and then another half a NoDoz pill in the midafternoon, when I tend to get sleepy. Then I sip sweet iced tea during the night. I sometimes drink Coca-Cola and Mountain Dew, but usually only during the day. You've got to know what works for you and stick to that during the race. Test out what works best for you during long-distance training days, so you are best prepared on race day.

Stage-Race Fueling

During the final race of the 4 Deserts Ultramarathon Series, Jax Mariash Mustafa opened her pack and pulled out her food stash for the night. Nutella, almonds, Fritos, and Endurox took up the most weight but contained the most calories per gram of fuel. Self-supported stage racing requires you to carry everything to survive on your back, including all your food for the weeklong journey ahead. It's an interesting balance between bringing the bare minimum to stay fueled for *optimal* performance and not bringing so much that your pack is too heavy. By the end, the pack is empty, and the athlete's goal is to maintain their weight (i.e., not lose too much). Jax lost 9 to 12 pounds during this weeklong stage race.

If you want to do multiple ultramarathon races at once, stage racing allows you to do just that. Stage races, which can be on foot or by bike, are particularly difficult to fuel for and recover from appropriately. Whether you have to carry all your own fuel for the entire event or you stop at the end of each day to refuel, it's crucial to replenish at least the bare minimum for the next day to keep yourself going.

- *Do a gradual carbohydrate increase before starting the stage race:* Start your gradual carbohydrate increase (7 to 12 grams per kilogram of body weight per day) three days before the start of the stage race. Focus on easily digestible carbohydrate sources (as mentioned in chapter 8).
- *Start each day off right:* Before a day of stage racing, make sure to get in a high amount of carbohydrates and calories to start off with plenty of fuel in your system. You will likely not be able to replenish your body completely at the end of each day, so managing your calorie deficit is important. Carbohydrate amounts before a stage day should equal one to two grams per kilogram of body weight of easily digested simple carb sources. Some protein and fat will keep you satiated, and you should tolerate them well going into the stage. Be sure to time your intake correctly, allowing yourself enough time to digest your meal, one to three hours before start time.
- *Hydrate, hydrate, hydrate:* It's important to hydrate before, during, and after each day of the stage race so you don't become too dehydrated during the full event. For many athletes, hydration can be an afterthought, especially after a long, hard day, but it is important to continue with a regular hydration routine at the end of each stage. Knowing your fluid loss rate before starting the stage race can help you gauge how much you need to consume every hour while you are moving.
- *Weigh yourself if possible:* If weighing yourself is a possibility at the start and end of each stage, it could help with your fluid replenishment targets. Aim to replace 20 to 24 ounces (600 to 720 milliliters) of fluids for every pound you have lost. Day-to-day weighing may not be as helpful because of glycogen depletion and overall weight loss due to energy deficits.
- *Be sure to use electrolytes:* Because you will be competing multiple days in a row, electrolyte depletion can become a real concern if you are not using supplements. During the stage, focus on your sodium intake, aiming for 300 to 600 milligrams per hour. When you're not moving, it

could be beneficial to take a varied electrolyte supplement that contains some of the other electrolytes lost in sweat (potassium, magnesium, calcium, and chloride), which you may have trouble replacing via food because of limited food choices along the route.

• *Take energy-dense foods:* While you still want to aim for at least 30 grams of carbohydrate intake every hour, you may consider carrying and eating more fat and protein throughout the stages—nut butters, trail mix, and candy bars work well. Not only will this help you pack in more calories overall, but it can also help keep you satiated throughout the day.

• *Take advantage of the recovery window:* Immediately after you finish each stage, focus on the recovery process. While it will be impossible to replace all your glycogen stores, consuming carbohydrates and protein right away can help start the glycogen resynthesis process and stop muscle protein breakdown. Depending on what fuel sources are available to you, liquid options such as juice and protein shakes may be the easiest way to get nutrition in as soon as you are done.

Ultra Stage-Racing Fueling Tips From Jax

1. Self-supported stage racing requires you to carry everything to survive on your back, including all your food for the weeklong journey ahead. It's an interesting balance between bringing the bare minimum to stay fueled for optimal performance and not bringing so much that your pack is too heavy. The minimum fuel carrying requirement for these races is 2,000 calories per day, and you must carry a total of 14,000 calories for the week. As you eat during the week, your pack gets lighter. In these races, you are not only running in extreme conditions with a heavy pack but also testing the very minimum and combination of macros that you can eat to survive, race well, and perform optimally. You must learn to optimize what you need and what works for you in these conditions.

2. It is important to maximize recovery by resting and refueling the body with a lot of calories. I always take on a little extra weight by bringing my protein powder and recovery mix because it helps me recover better.

3. Stage racing focuses more on calories per gram than overall calories. You consume a lot more fat during these races—foods such as almonds, macadamia nuts, Oreos, Fritos, and Nutella. All these foods contain a lot of calories for less weight.

4. Consider bringing one of your favorite foods with you, even if it takes up a little more weight. There is nothing like being in the middle of a stage race and taking a bite of your favorite food out there—a little piece of home to keep you going.

OCR Fueling

Spartan World Champion Nicole Mericle hasn't always had her fueling strategy for OCR racing polished. Muscle cramps plagued her at the beginning of her career, leaving her limping to the finish lines of her events. It wasn't until she started adding electrolytes to her fueling routine that she noticed a marked difference in performance, and the cramps dissipated.

Obstacle course racing, or OCR racing, has grown in popularity in the past decade. What started as physical and mental training to prepare for the military turned into a physical test of endurance for the average person in the form of a race. OCR racing today ranges from 5Ks to marathons and 24-hour events. Participants are required to complete tasks along the way, such as carrying a sandbag, climbing a rope wall, wading through mud, or jumping over barbed wire.

Due to the diversity of OCR races, nutritional fueling plans will vary depending on the duration of the event and the obstacles included. The races themselves require a good mix of physical endurance, strength, power, and agility.

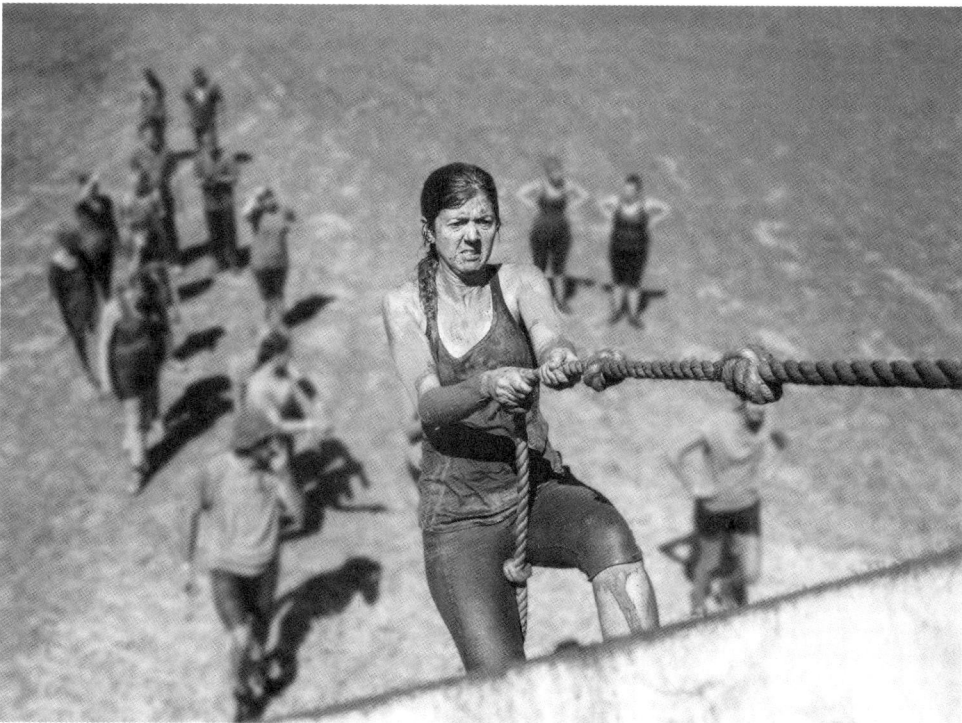

Jodie Griggs/The Image Bank RF/Getty Images

Nutrition fueling plans for obstacle course racing need to be personalized based on the race structure and duration.

Race Fueling Strategy

Because racing distances for these events vary, fueling strategies need to be personalized to optimize performance.

- For OCR events of less than 60 minutes, note the following:
  - Nutrition may not be realistic to carry and is technically not needed. It may benefit athletes who are racing shorter distances to ensure that they get a good prerace meal with one to two grams of carbohydrate per kilogram of body weight.
  - If the race will be hot or humid, consider taking in electrolytes with 16 to 20 ounces (480 to 600 milliliters) of fluids before the race.
  - You can take a gel in the 30 to 60 minutes before the gun goes off to give you an extra boost of energy throughout the race.
- For OCR events of more than 60 minutes, note the following:
  - Scope out aid stations ahead of time. Email the race director if you are having trouble finding what will be on the course.
  - For many OCR athletes, carrying nutrition can be logistically difficult. While some athletes may not mind wearing a hydration pack or waist belt for longer races, others may find it cumbersome to overcome obstacles while carrying their nutrition. If you're carrying nutrition products, make sure the packaging is easy to access and open, so you don't waste time on the course.

Nicole's Race-Day Tips

The biggest mistake I see people make is not fueling properly before and during races.

1. Many OCR events are quite early in the day, so it can be hard to wake up with enough time to eat a solid meal. It's also hard to force food down when you may not be hungry at 4:30 or 5:00 a.m., not to mention that race day nerves make it harder too. I go for foods that taste good to me—waffles with almond butter, berries, and some maple syrup—or try liquid calories that go down easier and quicker.

2. Races are deceivingly long, and athletes commonly underfuel as a result. For instance, a 13-mile training run takes way less time than a 13-mile run loaded with obstacles such as rope climbs and heavy carries. Looking at your previous race times helps you gauge your expected finish times and put together a realistic fueling schedule.

3. Setting an alarm also helps remind you when to take in fuel, especially if you find yourself getting distracted by obstacles.

- ◦ Relying on aid stations for fuel and hydration presents its own challenges—possibly improperly mixed hydration options, lack of allergen-free options, or a lack of diverse products that work for you.
- ◦ Keep in mind that because of the obstacles in the event, you need to time your nutrition choices appropriately (e.g., eating a whole cookie before going over an obstacle may not sit well). Save those gels and sports drinks for when you are about to hit the obstacles, and consider nibbling on solids at other times of the event.

Rowing-Specific Fueling

Rowers are unique athletes who train as endurance athletes but compete as sprinters. Due to the short duration of the races themselves, prerace nutrition is much more important for performance than nutrition during the race. However, if a rower chooses to take in fuel during competition or training, they should keep in mind the following tips:

- Easily digested carbohydrate sources like sports drinks and gels are preferrable. It is not advisable to use protein or fat as a fuel source during training or racing due to the high intensity and short duration of the races.
- You can use carbohydrate mouth rinses for a performance boost, even temporarily. Carbohydrate mouth rinses are theorized to stimulate taste receptors in the mouth, which activates neurons and can lead to enhanced performance. To perform a mouth rinse, an athlete rinses their mouth with a carbohydrate solution for 5 to 10 seconds, then spits it out. This strategy may be beneficial in training but may not be a practical technique during short races.

Fueling for Winter Sports (Cross-Country Skiing and Ski Mountaineering)

It was midnight on the night of the 2018 Grand Traverse ski mountaineering race from Crested Butte to Aspen. Skiers took a backcountry route throughout the night with the partner of their choice. Sean Van Horn, eventual winner of the event, took off with his partner, Cam Smith. The two of them skied into the night with temperatures dropping to 30 degrees Fahrenheit. A couple hours in, Sean went for a sip of water, but it was frozen, leaving him to ski with no hydration until the next aid station. Despite the fueling mishap, the team ended up making it to Aspen and skiing to victory.

Fueling for winter sports can be tricky and presents unique challenges. In cold temperatures, blood vessels constrict, sending blood to the core to keep us warm. This can diminish our thirst response. In addition, cold air tends to be drier. When we breathe it in, our lungs warm it and humidify it, and we lose extra fluids when we exhale. Sports nutrition products that we are used to using in the summer may freeze, and fluids may become undrinkable.

When we discuss endurance ski events, we are referencing two sports—cross-country skiing (which includes skate skiing and classic skiing) and ski mountaineering.

- *Cross-country skiing:* Cross-country skiing uses a lightweight ski in which the boot is fixed to the binding, but the heel is free. Skiers race across groomed snow over long distances. There are two main types of Nordic ski racing: skate skiing and classic skiing.

- *Ski mountaineering:* This ski event involves racing up and down mountainous terrain using specialized equipment—such as skins (think of little carpets for your skis)—and skinny, lightweight touring skis that allow the heel to float freely while going uphill and be fixed into a binding while going downhill.

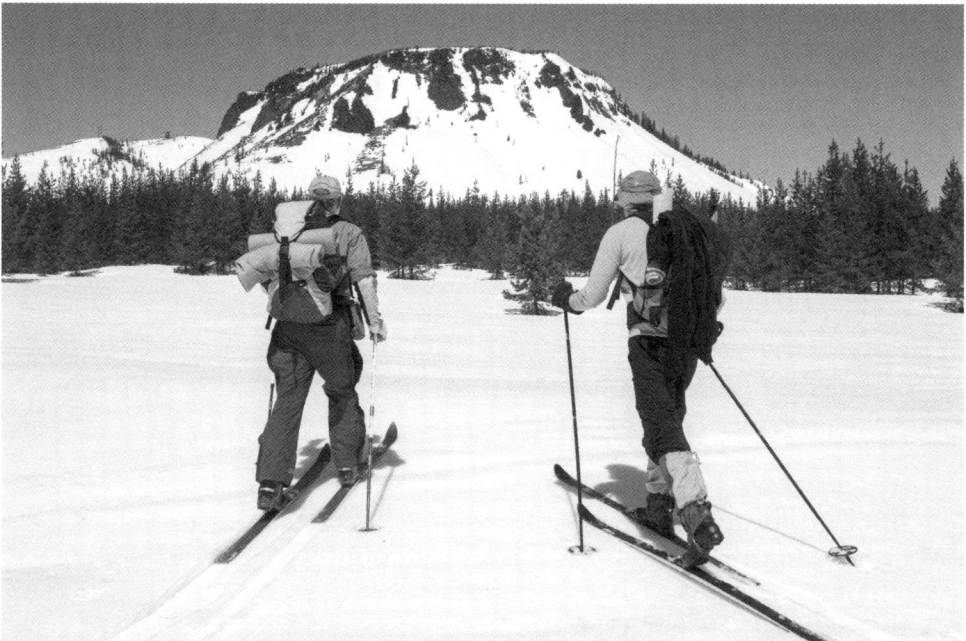

Cross-country skiing and other forms of ski racing provide unique challenges, but having a fueling plan in place with options will prepare you for event day.

Nutrition Targets During Cross-Country Skiing and Ski Mountaineering

For most of these races, you will need to rely on carbohydrates during exercise to power you through to the finish line. Aim to consume 30 to 90 grams of carbohydrate per hour. You may need to come up with creative strategies for consuming carbohydrates because you'll be holding on to poles while you're racing.

Even though it will likely be cold, you still need to replace lost fluids during these races. Figuring out your fluid loss rates in training will help you determine your target hourly fluid intake.

Tips for Eating and Drinking While Ski Racing

You will face unique challenges when ski racing, but the following shortcuts and tricks can help you plan your race fueling.

- Open prepackaged food (not gels!) ahead of time so you don't waste time or energy fumbling around to open them.
- Warm up your fluid before putting it in your bottles. Try to use insulated bottles or wrap a wool sock around your bottles to prevent freezing.
- Despite the cold, make sure you are drinking enough fluid throughout the race. To ensure your bottle valves and tubes do not freeze, blow air back into them after taking a drink.
- For longer ski mountaineering races, you may want to create your own insulated bladder suit you can hold close to your body to keep it from freezing.
- Pouring a small amount of vodka into your bladder suit can also prevent freezing.
- Test whether your food products will hold up to freezing by placing them in the freezer at home before going outside.
- You may need to consider different fueling options than you are used to due to the cold temperatures. Some sports gels may tolerate the cold, but many will freeze unless you keep them close to your body. Baked goods such as mini muffins, homemade protein balls, or and Stroop waffles may endure better and be easier to eat.

Takeaways

No matter the race durations you compete in as an endurance athlete, anticipate any sport-specific considerations so you can do the following:

- Fuel enough for the entire event, targeting appropriate macronutrient needs to keep yourself going with consistent energy and no gastrointestinal distress.
- Plan logistically for different sport-specific challenges regarding carrying, eating, and drinking enough.
- Have a backup plan(s) so you can adapt in case you are not able to follow the original fueling plan.

All race fueling strategies should be unique to the athlete and practiced extensively ahead of time to reduce the likelihood of a DNF. It might help to view your race fueling strategy as a way to gain an advantage over your opponents as you power through to the finish line.

10

POSTWORKOUT AND POSTRACE RECOVERY

A postworkout recovery beverage has been one of the biggest changes for me that has paid off dividends with my longevity and resilience in sport. I definitely lean on pretty traditional protein recovery drinks, most of which have at least some carbohydrate in them. This is because I have very busy days, and getting that in as soon as I'm done with my workout means I start that refueling and recovery phase immediately. Without this, I find myself running to class or a work meeting and not refueling properly for several hours [after] exercise. That and the tiniest bit of meal prepping means that I never go hungry [after a] workout and I never miss a meal.

—Corrine Malcolm, ex-professional Nordic skier and ultra-endurance athlete (athlete interview, 2022)

What would happen if, instead of focusing only on the endurance performance itself, you decided to also focus on all the little things that go into supporting your recovery afterward and your performance outside of that workout and race window?

A holistic recovery approach focuses not only on nutrition and nutrition timing but also on sleep, stress reduction, and self-care; it offers key opportunities to advance not only your performance but also your life. Such an approach can allow you to have longevity in the sports for which you push your body to its limits every day. The following sections will touch on each of these areas to help you holistically as an endurance athlete.

Postworkout Fueling

After a training session, your body relies on refueling to increase muscle protein synthesis, repair muscle fibers, and replenish glycogen stores. Eating the right composition and amount of fuel after exercise ensures your body is getting what it needs for these repair processes to happen effectively.

Endurance exercise depletes glycogen and amino acids, breaks down muscle fibers, and increases cellular damage. Postexercise nutrition composed of carbohydrates and protein gets the recovery process started. The idea of a "magical anabolic window of recovery" has been proposed, but this concept has been debated, and no recommendations on intake timing are definitive.

Concerning glycogen replenishment, it has been shown that glycogen depletion can increase muscle protein breakdown. When carbohydrate consumption is delayed by two hours after exercise, it can slow glycogen replenishment rates by up to 50 percent (Aragon and Schoenfeld 2013). Increased carbohydrate uptake rates immediately after exercise stem from increases in insulin-stimulated glucose uptake and glycogen synthase, which promotes carbohydrate storage.

Carbohydrates after exercise can provide quicker glycogen synthesis. Ingesting carbohydrates at the same time as protein may create better muscle protein synthesis rates, but the research results on this benefit are still mixed. This boost possibly stems from a more robust insulin response after exercise. Maximum glycogen replenishment rates have been achieved at a rate of 1 to 1.85 grams per kilogram per hour up to five hours after exercise (Jentjens and Jeukendrup 2003).

Muscle protein breakdown after exercise is slow at first but increases significantly with time after exercise has ceased (Aragon and Schoenfeld 2013). To achieve maximum rates of postexercise muscle protein synthesis, research supports taking in protein with or without carbohydrate rather than just carbohydrate alone. The maximum anabolic effect of postworkout protein is reached at an intake rate of 0.4 to 0.5 grams per pound or 20 to 40 grams of higher BCAA protein sources.

This information is seemingly only important for endurance athletes who rely on quick glycogen replenishment for their next training session, such as a triathlete performing two daily training sessions or an

Quick and Easy Postworkout Recovery Snacks

- 1 oz (30 g) jerky and 3 strips dried mango
- 1 cup (230 g) Greek yogurt with 1/2 cup (75 g) berries and 1/3 cup (35 g) granola
- PB&J sandwich and a protein shake with one scoop of protein powder
- Protein shake with one scoop of protein powder and a banana with 2 tbsp nut butter
- Protein-packed chia seed pudding with 1 tbsp honey and 1/2 cup (75 g) berries
- Sports recovery mix containing both carbohydrates and protein (common brands are Skratch Labs, Tailwind Nutrition, and GU Energy Labs)

endurance athlete doing an evening training session followed by an early-morning training session. However, this does not mean that focusing on postworkout nutrition and timing is not important.

For endurance athletes who want to optimize their recovery, it certainly can't hurt to get in the habit of including a regular postworkout snack that fits carbohydrate and protein guidelines in a timely manner. Athletes should consider their training duration, intensity, and frequency when determining the urgency of postworkout nutrition intake. The following suggestions are simple snack ideas that are great for recovery.

Postrace Nutrition

Though the event is finished, don't let your guard down after a long endurance race. Your glycogen stores are empty, and muscle protein and cellular damage is high. The goal of a postrace recovery plan is to replace your glycogen stores as quickly as possible—then you will be less sore, bounce back quickly, avoid sickness, and be able to function in daily life instead of just dragging yourself through the next day.

Postrace Recovery Plan

Having a postrace recovery plan ensures you are prepared after you complete your race without having to think about it—you can seamlessly make it happen. The following tips may help you anticipate potential challenges and identify what to focus on.

- *Anticipate a lack of appetite:* It's quite normal to lose your appetite after a long or hard effort due to alterations in hunger and fullness cues and in leptin and ghrelin (leptin, the fullness hormone, increases while ghrelin, the hunger hormone, decreases). Hormone changes can last the entire day or, worse yet, for days or weeks after ultra-endurance events. This can make it difficult to consume any kind of sustenance. Having liquid options available—recovery mixes, juices, soups, or smoothies—can be a great way to sip on some protein (20 grams of a high-quality option) and carbohydrates without feeling like you have to force yourself to chew or eat large amounts of food.

- *Get in fluids and electrolytes:* It's important to consume calories to replenish and repair, but many endurance athletes neglect to also get in fluids and electrolytes after a race. Bring an extra serving of electrolytes in your race bag so you don't have to go searching for them at the finish line area. Start with 250 to 500 milligrams of sodium in 16 ounces (480 milliliters) of fluids. Don't forget to replace more later in the day as you adjust back to normal. Remember, you'll need to replace all the sodium you didn't replace during exercise.

• *Eat a postrace recovery snack:* Consuming a postrace recovery snack within the first hour of finishing your race can speed up the glycogen replenishment process and slow or stop muscle protein breakdown. Have a snack packed in your bag for the finish line area so you don't have to think about it. Aim for 20 grams of high-quality protein and 1 to 2 grams per kilogram bodyweight of carbohydrate.

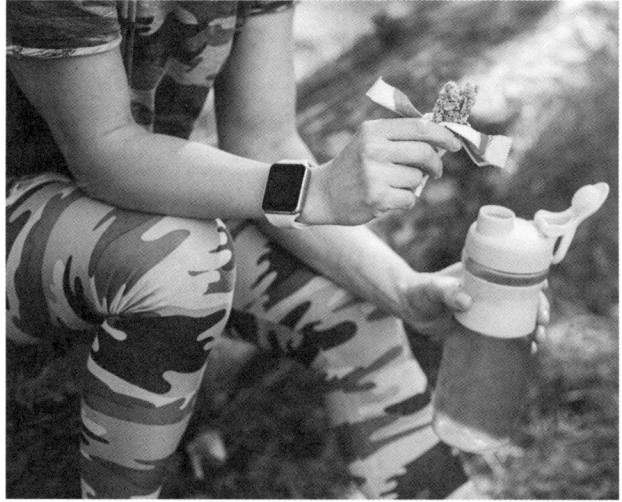

A protein bar and recovery drink are two options for postrace recovery fueling.

VlaDee/iStockphoto/Getty Images

• *Consider these packable postrace recovery snack options:*
  ○ Protein bar
  ○ Recovery mix (such as from Skratch Labs, Tailwind Nutrition, or GU Energy Labs)
  ○ Premixed nonperishable recovery shake (such as those from Orgain or OWYN)
  ○ PB&J with a nonperishable chocolate milk
  ○ Bagel with a nut or seed butter packet and a banana
  ○ Dried fruit pack and a meat stick or 1 oz (30 g) jerky

• *Choose your postrace beer carefully:* While many racers like to wind down with a postrace alcoholic beverage, remember that alcohol can inhibit glycogen replenishment and decrease muscle protein synthesis (Vella and Cameron-Smith 2010). If you are looking for nonalcoholic options, increasingly more companies are selling alternatives, or you can make your own with my favorite mocktail recipes, which follow.

• *Consider a massage:* Getting a postrace massage can really benefit endurance athletes. Massage itself can improve range of motion, lower swelling, and reduce pain. While manual massage therapy is preferred, you can also do self-massage or use compression tools.

The following are a few mocktail recipes to enjoy an alcohol-free celebration before or after the race. Cheers!

Sparkling Tart Cherry Lime

Ingredients

- 1/4 cup (60 mL) tart cherry juice
- 1 cup (240 mL) freshly squeezed orange juice (3 oranges)
- 1/4 cup (60 mL) lime juice
- 1/4 cup (60 mL) sparkling water

Directions

1. Pour tart cherry juice, orange juice, and lime juice into a pitcher and stir.
2. Divide into two cocktail glasses with ice and top with sparkling water.

Nonalcoholic Mojito

Ingredients

- 10 fresh mint leaves
- 3 lime wedges
- 2 tbsp granulated sugar
- 1/2 to 3/4 cup (120 to 180 mL) club soda

Directions

1. In a medium glass, muddle mint leaves and 1 lime wedge.
2. Muddle 2 more lime wedges and granulated sugar.
3. Fill cup with ice and top with club soda.
4. Garnish with more mint or lime wedges for a fun touch.

Coconut Cooler

Ingredients

- 4 cups (960 mL) coconut water
- 2 thinly sliced cucumbers
- 1/2 cup (120 mL) lime juice
- 1/4 cup (60 g) chopped mint leaves
- 1/4 cup (50 g) sugar (optional)

Directions

1. Combine coconut water, cucumbers, lime juice, mint leaves, and sugar (optional). Stir.
2. Let chill for 1 to 2 hours and serve.

Watermelon Mock Margarita

Ingredients

- 4 cups (640 g) seedless watermelon
- 1/2 cup (120 mL) fresh lime juice
- 4 tsp agave
- Sparkling water (to top off cups)

Directions

1. Use a blender to puree watermelon.
2. Add lime juice and agave and blend again.
3. Pour into four cups and top with sparkling water.

How to Eat the Week After Your Race to Optimize Recovery

Figuring out how to eat the week after a race can be a stressful experience for endurance athletes. During the recovery process, the body is desperately trying to replenish lost glycogen stores, repair broken-down muscle fibers, and reregulate its physiological systems. Excess postexercise oxygen consumption (EPOC) occurs because of an increase in exercise intensity and affects oxygen consumption and metabolism. EPOC typically results in increased heart rate, elevated hormones, elevated neurotransmitters, increased respiration, and elevated core temperature. Because of EPOC, it is important to keep in mind that even though you might be resting after a race, your metabolism may stay elevated for many days to aid in this recovery process. Decreasing energy intake drastically for fear of weight gain can backfire on athletes and increase the risk of injury or illness. For many athletes, this can alter hunger and fullness feelings and increase cravings for carbohydrates and protein. If your appetite is suppressed, remember that your body still needs additional nutrition to recover.

Easy Recovery Meals When You Have No Appetite

- 2-3 slices of pizza with a protein shake (to get a protein boost)
- 3 eggs with 1 cup (230 g) white rice and half an avocado
- Fruit smoothie bowl with granola, coconut, and fruit as toppings
- 1-1/2 cups (345 g) chili (with or without meat) topped with 1 oz (30 g) cheese and a side of French bread
- Loaded avocado toast: 2 slices of sourdough bread, 2 slices of bacon, 1 avocado, and 2 eggs
- Loaded nachos: tortilla chips topped with your choice of protein (2/3 cup [160 g] beans or 4 oz [115 g] meat), cheese (however much

you like), half an avocado, 1/2 cup (115 g) salsa (optional), and sour cream (optional)

- Macaroni and cheese with 4 oz (115 g) meat or tofu added for protein and 8 oz (240 mL) juice on the side
- Plain buttered noodles with a 4 oz (115 g) chicken breast or meat alternative

Postworkout Recovery Recipes by Kelly Newlon of RAD in Boulder, Colorado

Cornbread and Beans Bake

This recipe is made in a pan and can be cooled, cut, and wrapped in individual portions to pull out and heat up. This dish is super easy to make with many variations, and it's great to eat after a workout. Baked layers of carbohydrates, proteins, and a bit of fiber and micronutrients provide all the things you need to recover quickly.

Note: This is also a great option for crews or pacers to take to long overnight races so they have something to eat while helping the athletes.

Ingredients
- 2/3 cup (153 g) butter or butter alternative
- 1/2 (100 g) cup brown sugar
- 3 eggs (or 3/4 cup [480 mL] Just Egg)
- 1-2/3 cup (400 mL) milk or milk alternative
- 1-1/3 cup (200 g) cornmeal
- 2 cups (240 g) flour or gluten-free flour
- 1-1/2 tbsp baking powder
- 1/2 tsp kosher salt
- 1 cup (180 g) cooked beans (a combination of black and white beans is great)

Directions
1. Preheat oven to 350 °F (177 °C).
2. Use a 9 x 13 in. (27 x 39 cm) pan for a double recipe. We use a 9-in. cast-iron pan for this recipe at home.
3. Add everything to a large bowl and mix until just incorporated.
4. Pour into the greased pan and bake until set, about 45 minutes.
5. Cool, cut, and wrap in individual squares. Can be frozen for up to two months.

Professional Chef/Sports Nutrition.

Chorizo and Chickpeas

This is a quick sauté that is easily made vegan if necessary. Adding an egg on top is a great way to get in more protein. It can be eaten as is or rolled into a tortilla to get more carbohydrates.
Servings: 2

Ingredients

- 1 lb (460 g) chorizo or plant-based chorizo
- 1 can cooked chickpeas
- 1/4 cup (60 mL) water
- 1 cup (150 g) cherry tomatoes
- 1/4 cup (6 g) fresh chopped basil
- 1/4 cup (31 g) goat cheese or plant-based goat or feta cheese

Directions

1. In a large sauté pan, cook the chorizo on medium heat until fully cooked. Be sure to stir it while it cooks to prevent burning and break the chorizo into pieces. Chorizo has a bit of fat in it already, so I don't add fat to this recipe, but feel free to add 2 tbsp of olive oil if desired.
2. Once the chorizo is done, add chickpeas, tomatoes, and water.
3. Stir to combine and cook for 1 minute.
4. Turn the burner off and add basil and cheese.
5. Mix thoroughly and enjoy!

Professional Chef/Sports Nutrition.

Injured Athlete Nutrition

What happens if you get injured? The last thing an endurance athlete wants to deal with is an injury that takes them out of training and racing for months on end. Whether it's a bone stress injury or a ligament or tendon issue, this becomes the question: Can you really eat your way to recovery? Prioritizing nutrition as a tool to aid in the recovery process can help maintain muscle mass and inflammation levels—not to mention that nutrition can help you heal the fastest and return to competition.

- *Energy requirements:* It might be tempting to significantly decrease your energy intake when injury strikes because of reduced physical activity. However, to support healing, your metabolism may be slightly elevated, at least initially, after an injury. Don't restrict intake too much because an energy deficit can accelerate muscle loss.

• *Protein:* It may be particularly advantageous to increase protein consumption to 2.0 (and no less than 1.6) grams per kilogram of body weight per day, even with a slight reduction in overall energy intake, because you'll typically have longer periods of immobility, a lack of muscle contraction, and a lack of weight-bearing. Aim for regular intake windows for meals and snacks every day. High-quality (BCAA) protein sources that are rich in leucine can support the highest rates of muscle protein synthesis throughout the recovery process (see table 10.1; USDA Food Data Central, 2024).

• *Carbohydrates:* While carbohydrates are still important for normal body function and energy production, they may not be as necessary throughout the injury recovery process. They can also negate a catabolic state.

• *Antioxidants:* While some inflammation is a good thing, consuming antioxidant-rich foods—including tart cherry juice, pomegranate juice, turmeric, ginger, dark chocolate (more than 70 percent cacao), green tea (rich in epigallocatechin gallate [EGCG]), and assorted colors of fruits and vegetables—provides additional support to keep inflammation in check.

TABLE 10.1 Foods Highest in BCAA Content

Food	Portion	Amount of BCAAs
Whey protein powder	1 scoop	5.9 g
Chicken breast	3.5 oz (100 g)	5.5 g
Ground beef	3.5 oz (100g)	4.5 g
Salmon	3.5 oz (100 g)	4.0 g
Eggs	2 whole	2.6 g
Milk	8 oz (240 mL)	1.7 g
Greek yogurt	1/2 cup (115 g)	2.0 g

Source: USDA Foods Database.

Other Recovery Considerations

Rest, relaxation, and self-care can sometimes seem like foreign ideas to endurance athletes who are always on the go. But with all the stress you put your body under during endurance events, it is important to prioritize other recovery modalities to keep you in balance. Sleep, foam rolling, yoga, meditation, stress reduction, massage, and acupuncture are all ways to effectively help the body rebound, repair, and rejuvenate so you can come back stronger.

Sleep Needs

While you may not sleep the best right after your race, prioritizing sleep in the days and weeks following your event is one of the best ways to recover. Research clearly shows that increasing the duration and quality of sleep is one of the best ways to increase performance and mental well-being after a race (Samuels and James 2014).

Sleep duration and quality are the most important factors when looking at benefits for endurance athletes. Unfortunately, sleep is often neglected by endurance athletes with busy training schedules, life responsibilities, and intruding technology (computers and cell phones). All endurance athletes should regularly evaluate their sleep quality and duration as it relates to their training and construct an optimized sleep routine. Using earplugs, eye masks, and blackout curtains can make the bedroom more conducive to better quality sleep.

Lack of sleep can lead to the following:

- Reduction in performance
- Reduction in decision-making ability
- Reduction in learning and cognition
- Reduction in immune function
- Reduction in tissue repair capabilities
- Changes in glucose and neuroendocrine function, which in turn can affect carbohydrate metabolism, appetite, food intake, and protein synthesis

An effective sleep routine could include the following:

- Keep a sleep diary with information on bedtime, wake-up time, and total sleep time to gain insight into your sleep habits.
- Keep your room dark. Blackout curtains or an eye mask can block out light and prevent it from interfering with your rest. Let in bright light in the morning to wake your body up.
- Try tart cherry juice! It's a natural source of melatonin, so a serving one hour before bedtime can promote sleep.
- Be careful when you nap! Napping too long or too late in the day can throw off your sleep schedule.
- Pick a bedtime and a wake-up time and stick to them as closely as you can, even on the weekends. This can help your body get accustomed to a healthy sleep routine.
- Try to stay off any electronic devices 30 minutes before going to bed because the light from screens can suppress your natural melatonin production. Aim to do quiet, calm activities before bedtime (such as reading or listening to soothing music) instead.

- Have a high-protein snack before bed to promote sleep and recovery.
- Keep an eye on your caffeine intake; using caffeine to overcome daytime sleepiness can cause long-term sleep deprivation. Do not consume it later in the day because this can be a barrier to falling asleep at night.
- Doing the same things every night before you go to sleep, such as taking a shower or reading a book, can signal to your body that it is time for bed.

Stress Reduction

Lowering stress by reducing commitments and avoiding overexertion in the weeks following your race can aid in appropriate recovery. Developing daily stress-reduction and self-care routines can ensure you are managing stressors outside of your training stress to avoid burnout and fatigue. Trying stress-reduction techniques such as deep breathing, yoga, or meditation and engaging in self-care activities such as soaking in the bathtub or getting a massage can encourage you to slow down and give your body time to restore and repair itself. It is important to choose nutrition, sleep, and stress-reduction routines that respect your body and lifestyle.

Takeaways

Throughout this book, you'll notice a theme. The approach used here is not focused on restriction or rules. There are no fads, hacks, or gimmicks—no focus on weight loss, body composition, or manipulation of your body with less fuel. The focus is placed on the whole endurance athlete and is set up to help you thrive, not just survive, by condensing a confusing mass of nutrition information into a practical nutrition guide.

Why? When you start focusing on optimizing and stop restricting, that's where the magic happens. When you don't fully give your body what it needs, you risk losing all the adaptations you could be getting from your training, increase the risk of injury and illness, and push your mind into obsession. While some endurance athletes might have success manipulating their diet to extremes, that is not the norm. Remember, if it sounds too good to be true, it probably is.

In my work with thousands of endurance athletes, I've found the following to be true. I present these statements to you so you can make the best choices for the future of your endurance body and mind.

- It's important to follow a nutrition plan that works for your lifestyle, not someone else's.

- Being overly prepared with your race fueling strategy is key. Practice, practice, practice. Make contingency plans, and predict that things will go wrong. Plan to have to adapt in the moment.

- Using weight and body composition as your only motivators for performance gains will lead you down a path of obsession and misery. Do you really want to be tied to numbers and vanity metrics for the rest of your life? Remember, endurance athletes don't look a certain way.

- Plan ahead. Some level of planning is required for you to succeed at fueling yourself to the necessary extent. Carve out time each week and make it happen, no matter what.

- Hydration and electrolytes are often-overlooked tools that can improve fatigue levels.

- Prioritize sleep and rest just as much as training and nutrition. Exercising more and pushing harder is not the boast you might think it is.

- Supplement wisely. There is no need to blindly supplement with no reasons behind what you are doing. Check your blood work. Understand why you are using something. Use reputable supplement companies.

- Be skeptical of quick fixes and extreme diets. Carbs are good.

- Having optimized preworkout and postworkout recovery plans can make all the difference for your next workout or race.

- Don't underestimate the power of listening to your body's hunger and fullness cues. If you don't know what that looks like for you, take the time to understand what hunger and fullness feel like. Journal, take notes, and be mentally present when fueling yourself.

Take this book as a guide and use it as you see fit. My hope is that it will open your eyes to a new perspective on endurance fueling—one that pushes the fueling limits. No matter what endurance path you find yourself on, always remember this: Fuel often. Fuel enough. Fuel intentionally.

REFERENCES

CHAPTER 1

Baker, J.S., M.C. McCormick, and R.A. Robergs. 2010. "Interaction Among Skeletal Muscle Metabolic Energy Systems During Intense Exercise." *Journal of Nutrition and Metabolism* 2010, 905612. https://doi.org/10.1155/2010/905612.

Douglas, J.A., J.A. King, E. McFarlane, L. Baker, C. Bradley, N. Crouch, D. Hill, and D.J. Stensel. 2015. "Appetite, Appetite Hormone and Energy Intake Responses to Two Consecutive Days of Aerobic Exercise in Healthy Young Men." *Appetite* 92:57-65. https://doi.org/10.1016/j.appet.2015.05.006.

Fensham, N.C., I.A. Heikura, A.K.A McKay, N. Tee, K.E. Ackerman, and L.M. Burke. 2022. "Short-Term Carbohydrate Restriction Impairs Bone Formation at Rest and During Prolonged Exercise to a Greater Degree Than Low Energy Availability." *Journal of Bone and Mineral Research* 37 (10): 1915-1925. https://doi.org/10.1002/jbmr.4658.

Fuller, D., E. Colwell, J. Low, K. Orychock, M.A. Tobin, B. Simango, R. Buote, D. Van Heerden, H. Luan, K. Cullen, L. Slade, and N.G.A Taylor. 2020. "Reliability and Validity of Commercially Available Wearable Devices for Measuring Steps, Energy Expenditure, and Heart Rate: Systematic Review.: *JMIR mHealth and uHealth* 8 (9): e18694. https://doi.org/10.2196/18694.

Hurford, M. 2016. "Timeline: A History of Tour de France Nutrition." *Bicycling*. July 22, 2016. www.bicycling.com/health-nutrition/a20040926/timeline-a-history-of-tour-de-france-nutrition/.

Melin, A., Å.B. Tornberg, S. Skouby, S.S. Møller, J. Sundgot-Borgen, J. Faber, J.J. Sidelmann, M. Aziz, and A. Sjödin. 2015. "Energy Availability and the Female Athlete Triad in Elite Endurance Athletes." *Scandinavian Journal of Medicine and Science in Sports* 25 (5): 610-22. https://doi.org/10.1111/sms.12261.

Mountjoy, M., K.E. Ackerman, D.M. Bailey, L.M. Burke, N. Constantini, A.C. Hackney, I.A. Heikura et al. 2023. "2023 International Olympic Committee's (IOC) Consensus Statement on Relative Energy Deficiency in Sport (REDs)." *British Journal of Sports Medicine* 57 (17): 1073-97. https://doi.org./10.1136/bjsports-2023-106994. Erratum in: *British Journal of Sports Medicine* 58 (3): e4.

Murakami, K., and M.B.E. Livingstone. 2015. "Prevalence and Characteristics of Misreporting of Energy Intake in US Adults: NHANES 2003-2012." *British Journal of Nutrition* 114 (8): 1294-303. https://doi.org/10.1017/S0007114515002706.

Rapp, J., A. Tierney, H. Frazee, D. Skinner, K. Smith, E. Sedjo, K. Jackson, and N. Anderson. 2021. "Optimizing Sport Performance by Looking Beyond Weight." McCallum Place Eating Disorders Centers. May 21, 2021. www.mccallumplace.com/about/blog/optimizing-sport-performance/.

Robinson, R. 2010. "Marathon Fueling Fumbles From the Past." *Runner's World*. March 30, 2010. www.runnersworld.com/advanced/a20789765/marathon-fueling-fumbles-from-the-past/.

Tribole, E. and Resch, E. (1995) *Intuitive Eating: A Revolutionary Program That Works.* Saint Martin's Paperbacks, New York.

CHAPTER 2

Abbasi, B., M. Kimiagar, K. Sadeghniiat, M.M. Shirazi, M. Hedayati, and B. Rashid-khani. 2012. "The Effect of Magnesium Supplementation on Primary Insomnia in Elderly: A Double-Blind Placebo-Controlled Clinical Trial." *Journal of Research in Medical Sciences* 17 (12): 1161-69.

Academy of Nutrition and Dietetics. 2018. "High Iron List of Foods Handout."

Bakian, A.V., R.S. Huber, L. Scholl, P.F. Renshaw, and D. Kondo. 2020. "Dietary Creatine Intake and Depression Risk Among U.S. Adults." *Translational Psychiatry* 10, 52. https://doi.org/10.1038/s41398-020-0741-x.

Beard, J., & Tobin, B. (2000). Iron status and exercise. *The American journal of clinical nutrition*, 72(2 Suppl), 594S–7S.

Berkheiser, K. 2023. "How Much Magnesium Should You Take Per Day?" Healthline. Last modified November 13, 2023. www.healthline.com/nutrition/magnesium-dosage.

Brittenham, G.M. 2018. "Disorders of Iron Homeostasis: Iron Deficiency and Overload." In *Hematology: Basic Principles and Practice*, 7th ed., edited by R. Hoffman, E.J. Benz, L.E. Silberstein, H.E. Heslop, J.I. Weitz, J. Anastasi, M.E. Salama, and S.A. Abutalib, 478-90. Philadelphia: Elsevier. https://doi.org/10.1016/B978-0-323-35762-3.00036-6.

Cerqueira, É., D.A. Marinho, H.P. Neiva, and O. Lourenço. 2020. "Inflammatory Effects of High and Moderate Intensity Exercise—A Systematic Review." *Frontiers in Physiology* 10, 1550. https://doi.org/10.3389/fphys.2019.01550.

Córdova, A., J. Mielgo-Ayuso, E. Roche, A. Caballero-García, and D. Fernandez-Lázaro. 2019. "Impact of Magnesium Supplementation in Muscle Damage of Professional Cyclists Competing in a Stage Race." *Nutrients* 11 (8): 1927. https://doi.org/10.3390/nu11081927.

Cox, P., T. Kirk, T. Ashmore, K. Willerton, R. Evans, A. Smith, A.J. Murray et al. 2016. "Nutritional Ketosis Alters Preference and Thereby Endurance Performance in Athletes." *Cell Metabolism* 24 (2): P256-68. https://doi.org/10.1016/j.cmet.2016.07.010.

Dawson, B., C. Goodman, T. Blee, G. Claydon, P. Peeling, J. Beilby, and A. Prins. 2006. "Iron Supplementation: Oral Tablets Versus Intramuscular Injection." *International Journal of Sport Nutrition and Exercise Metabolism* 16 (2): 180-86. https://doi.org/10.1123/ijsnem.16.2.180.

Doherty, M., and P.M. Smith. 2005. "Effects of Caffeine Ingestion on Rating of Perceived Exertion During and After Exercise: A Meta-Analysis." *Scandinavian Journal of Medicine and Science in Sports* 15 (2): 69-78. https://doi.org/10.1111/j.1600-0838.2005.00445.x.

Drobnic, F., F. Rueda, V. Pons, M. Banquells, B. Cordobilla, and J.C. Domingo. 2017. "Erythrocyte Omega-3 Fatty Acid Content in Elite Athletes in Response to Omega-3 Supplementation: A Dose-Response Pilot Study." *Journal of Lipids* 2017, 1472719. https://doi.org/10.1155/2017/1472719.

Evans, M., T.S. McClure, A.P. Koutnik, and B. Egan. 2022. "Exogenous Ketone Supplements in Athletic Contexts: Past, Present, and Future." *Sports Medicine* 52 (Suppl 1): 25-67. https://doi.org/10.1007/s40279-022-01756-2.

Guest, N.S., T.A. VanDusseldorp, M.T. Nelson, J. Grgic, B.J. Schoenfeld, N.D.M. Jenkins, S.M. Arent et al. 2021. "International Society of Sports Nutrition Position Stand: Caffeine and Exercise Performance." *Journal of the International Society of Sports Nutrition* 18 (1). https://doi.org/10.1186/s12970-020-00383-4.

Harris, R.C., G. Jones, and J.A. Wise. 2008. "The Plasma Concentration-Time Profile of Beta-Alanine Using a Controlled-Release Formulation (Carnosyn ®)." *The FASEB Journal* 22 (S1). https://doi.org/10.1096/fasebj.22.1_supplement.701.9.

Heaton, L.E., J.K. Davis, E.S. Rawson, R.P. Nuccio, O.C. Witard, K.W. Stein, K. Baar, J.M. Carter, and L.B. Baker. 2017. "Selected In-Season Nutritional Strategies to Enhance Recovery for Team Sport Athletes: A Practical Overview." *Sports Medicine* 47 (11): 2201-18. https://doi.org/10.1007/s40279-017-0759-2.

Hobson, R.M., B. Saunders, G. Ball, R.C. Harris, and C. Sale. 2012. "Effects of β-Alanine Supplementation on Exercise Performance: A Meta-Analysis." *Amino Acids* 43:25-37. https://doi.org/10.1007/s00726-011-1200-z.

Holick, M.F., N.C. Binkley, H.A. Bischoff-Ferrari, C.M. Gordon, D.A. Hanley, R.P. Heaney, M.H. Murad, and C.M. Weaver. 2011. "Evaluation, Treatment, and Prevention of Vitamin D Deficiency: An Endocrine Society Clinical Practice Guideline." *Journal of Clinical Endocrinology and Metabolism* 96 (7): 1911-30. https://doi.org/10.1210/jc.2011-0385.

Hormoznejad, R., A.Z. Javid, and A. Mansoori. 2019. "Effect of BCAA Supplementation on Central Fatigue, Energy Metabolism Substrate and Muscle Damage to the Exercise: A Systematic Review with Meta-Analysis." *Sport Sciences for Health* 15:265-79. https://doi.org/10.1007/s11332-019-00542-4.

Jensen, N.S., M. Wehland, P.M. Wise, and D. Grimm. 2023. "Latest Knowledge on the Role of Vitamin D in Hypertension." *International Journal of Molecular Sciences* 24 (5): 4679. https://doi.org/10.3390/ijms24054679.

Kreider, R.B., D.S. Kalman, J. Antonio, T.N. Ziegenfuss, R. Wildman, R. Collins, D.G. Candow, S.M. Kleiner, A.L. Almada, and H.L. Lopez. 2017. "International Society of Sports Nutrition Position Stand: Safety and Efficacy of Creatine Supplementation in Exercise, Sport, and Medicine." *Journal of the International Society of Sports Nutrition* 14 (1). https://doi.org/10.1186/s12970-017-0173-z.

Lara, B., C. Ruiz-Moreno, J.J. Salinero, and J. Del Coso. 2019. "Time Course of Tolerance to the Performance Benefits of Caffeine." *PLoS ONE* 14 (1): e0210275. https://doi.org/10.1371/journal.pone.0210275.

Macuh, M., and B. Knap. 2021. "Effects of Nitrate Supplementation on Exercise Performance in Humans: A Narrative Review." *Nutrients* 13 (9): 3183. https://doi.org/10.3390/nu13093183.

Mathews, N.M. 2018. "Prohibited Contaminants in Dietary Supplements." *Sports Health* 10 (1): 19-30. https://doi.org/10.1177/1941738117727736.

McCormick, R., M. Sim, B. Dawson, and P. Peeling. 2020. "Refining Treatment Strategies for Iron Deficient Athletes." *Sports Medicine* 50:2111-23. https://doi.org/10.1007/s40279-020-01360-2.

Mignon, P. 2003. "The Tour de France and the Doping Issue." *International Journal of the History of Sport* 20 (2): 227-45. https://doi.org/10.1080/09523360412331305703.

Miller, J.R., K.W. Dunn, L.J. Ciliberti, Jr., R.D. Patel, and B.A. Swanson. 2016. "Association of Vitamin D With Stress Fractures: A Retrospective Cohort Study." *Journal of Foot and Ankle Surgery* 55 (1): 117-20. https://doi.org/10.1053/j.jfas.2015.08.002.

National Institutes of Health. 2021. "Magnesium: Fact Sheet for Consumers." Last modified March 22, 2021. https://ods.od.nih.gov/factsheets/Magnesium-Consumer/.

Nelson, A.G., D.A. Arnall, J. Kokkonen, R. Day, and J. Evans. 2001. "Muscle Glycogen Supercompensation Is Enhanced by Prior Creatine Supplementation." *Medicine and Science in Sports and Exercise* 33 (7): 1096-100. https://doi.org/10.1097/00005768-200107000-00005.

Nielsen, F.H., and H.C. Lukaski. 2006. "Update on the Relationship Between Magnesium and Exercise." *Magnesium Research* 19 (3): 180-89.

Nutrition Business Journal. 2017. *Supplement Business Report 2016*. New York: Penton.

Office of Dietary Supplements. (2022, March 26). Omega-3 fatty acids: Fact sheet for health professionals. National Institutes of Health. https://ods.od.nih.gov/factsheets/Omega3FattyAcids-HealthProfessional/

Philpott, J.D., O.C. Witard, and S.D.R. Galloway. 2019. "Applications of Omega-3 Polyunsaturated Fatty Acid Supplementation for Sport Performance." *Research in Sports Medicine* 27 (2): 219-37. https://doi.org/10.1080/15438627.2018.1550401.

Poffé, C., M. Ramaekers, S. Bogaerts, and P. Hespel. 2021. "Bicarbonate Unlocks the Ergogenic Action of Ketone Monoester Intake in Endurance Exercise." *Medicine and Science in Sports and Exercise* 53 (2): 431-41. https://doi.org/10.1249/MSS.0000000000002467.

Poffé, C., M. Ramaekers, R. Van Thienen, and P. Hespel. 2019. "Ketone Ester Supplementation Blunts Overreaching Symptoms During Endurance Training Overload." *Journal of Physiology* 597 (12): 3009-27. https://doi.org/10.1113/JP277831.

Poffé, C., R. Robberechts, M. Stalmans, J. Vanderroost, S. Bogaerts, and P. Hespel. 2023. "Exogenous Ketosis Increases Circulating Dopamine Concentration and Maintains Mental Alertness in Ultra-Endurance Exercise." *Journal of Applied Physiology* 134 (6): 1456-69. https://doi.org/10.1152/japplphysiol.00791.2022.

Reno, A.M., M. Green, L.G. Killen, E.K. O'Neal, K. Pritchett, and Z. Hanson. 2022. "Effects of Magnesium Supplementation on Muscle Soreness and Performance." *Journal of Strength and Conditioning Research* 36 (8): 2198-203. https://doi.org/10.1519/JSC.0000000000003827.

Rokkedal-Lausch, T., J. Franch, M.K. Poulsen, L.P. Thomsen, E. Weitzberg, E.N. Kamavuako, D.S. Karbing, and R.G. Larsen. 2019. "Chronic High-Dose Beetroot Juice Supplementation Improves Time Trial Performance of Well-Trained Cyclists in Normoxia and Hypoxia." *Nitric Oxide* 85:44-52. https://doi.org/10.1016/j.niox.2019.01.011.

Santos, R.V.T., R.A Bassit, E.C. Caperuto, and L.F.B.P. Costa Rosa. 2004. "The Effect of Creatine Supplementation on Inflammatory and Muscle Soreness Markers After a 30KM Race." *Life Sciences* 75 (16): 1917-24. https://doi.org/10.1016/j.lfs.2003.11.036.

Schuchardt, J.P., and A. Hahn. 2013. "Bioavailability of Long-Chain Omega-3 Fatty Acids." *Prostaglandins, Leukotrienes and Essential Fatty Acids* 89 (1): 1-8. https://doi.org/10.1016/j.plefa.2013.03.010.

Sim, M., L.A. Garvican-Lewis, G.R. Cox, A. Govus, A.K.A. McKay, T. Stellingwerff, and P. Peeling. 2019. "Iron Considerations for the Athlete: A Narrative Review." *European Journal of Applied Physiology* 119:1463-78. https://doi.org/10.1007/s00421-019-04157-y.

Sonneville, K.R., C.M. Gordon, M.S. Kocher, L.M. Pierce, A. Ramappa, and A.E. Field. 2012. "Vitamin D, Calcium, and Dairy Intakes and Stress Fractures Among Female Adolescents." *Archives of Pediatrics and Adolescent Medicine* 166 (7): 595-600. https://doi.org/10.1001/archpediatrics.2012.5.

Southward, K., K.J. Rutherfurd-Markwick, and A. Ali. 2018. "The Effect of Acute Caffeine Ingestion on Endurance Performance: A Systematic Review and Meta-Analysis." *Sports Medicine* 48:1913-28. https://doi.org/10.1007/s40279-018-0939-8.

Stout, J., J. Eckerson, K. Ebersole, G. Moore, S. Perry, T. Housh, A. Bull, J. Cramer, and A. Batheja. 2000. "Effect of Creatine Loading on Neuromuscular Fatigue Threshold." *Journal of Applied Physiology* 88 (1): 109-12. https://doi.org/10.1152/jappl.2000.88.1.109.

Stubbs, B.J., P.J. Cox, T. Kirk, R.D. Evans, and K. Clarke. 2019. "Gastrointestinal Effects of Exogenous Ketone Drinks are Infrequent, Mild, and Vary According to Ketone Compound and Dose." *International Journal of Sport Nutrition and Exercise Metabolism* 29 (6): 596-603. https://doi.org/10.1123/ijsnem.2019-0014.

Sung, C.C., M.T. Liao, K.C. Lu, and C.C. Wu. 2012. "Role of Vitamin D in Insulin Resistance." *Journal of Biomedicine and Biotechnology* 2012, 634195. https://doi.org/10.1155/2012/634195.

University of Oxford. 2016. "Ketone Drink Gives Competitive Cyclists a Boost by Altering Their Metabolism." July 29, 2016. www.ox.ac.uk/news/2016-07-29-ketone-drink-gives-competitive-cyclists-boost-altering-their-metabolism.

U.S. Anti-Doping Agency. n.d. "Independence and History." Accessed August 24, 2024. www.usada.org/independence-history/.

U.S. Congress. 1994. "S.784 - Dietary Supplement Health and Education Act of 1994." October 25, 1994. www.congress.gov/bill/103rd-congress/senate-bill/784.

U.S. Department of Agriculture. 2015. "USDA National Nutrient Database for Standard Reference: Release 28." Oct 19, 2015. https://ods.od.nih.gov/pubs/usdandb/VitaminD-Content.pdf.

Wacker, M., and M.F. Holick. 2013. "Vitamin D—Effects on Skeletal and Extraskeletal Health and the Need for Supplementation." *Nutrients* 5 (1): 111-48. https://doi.org/10.3390/nu5010111.

World Anti-Doping Agency. (n.d.). Prohibited list. Accessed on August 24, 2024 https://www.wada-ama.org/en/prohibited-list.

CHAPTER 3

Baker, L.B. 2017. "Sweating Rate and Sweat Sodium Concentration in Athletes: A Review of Methodology and Intra/Interindividual Variability." *Sports Medicine* 47 (Suppl 1): 111-28. https://doi.org/10.1007/s40279-017-0691-5.

Bouscaren, N., G.Y. Millet, and S. Racinais. 2019. "Heat Stress Challenges in Marathon vs. Ultra-Endurance Running." *Frontiers in Sports and Active Living* 1, 59. https://doi.org/10.3389/fspor.2019.00059.

Butterfield, G.E., J. Gates, S. Fleming, G.A. Brooks, J.R. Sutton, and J.T. Reeves. 1992. "Increased Energy Intake Minimizes Weight Loss in Men at High Altitude." *Journal of Applied Physiology* 72 (5): 1741-48. https://doi.org/10.1152/jappl.1992.72.5.1741.

Gopathi, P., K.H. Tiwari, and K. Kalpana. 2023. "The Effects of Pre-Exercise Ice-Slurry Ingestion on Thermoregulation and Exercise Performance of Highly Trained Athletes: A Scoping Review." *International Journal of Exercise Science* 16 (2): 1398-1412.

Govus, A.D., L.A. Garvican-Lewis, C.R. Abbiss, P. Peeling, and C.J. Gore. 2015. "Pre-Altitude Serum Ferritin Levels and Daily Oral Iron Supplement Dose Mediate Iron Parameter and Haemoglobin Mass Responses to Altitude Exposure." *PLoS ONE* 10 (8): e0135120. https://doi.org/10.1371/journal.pone.0135120.

Maughan, R.J., and S.M. Shirreffs. 2019. "Muscle Cramping During Exercise: Causes, Solutions, and Questions Remaining." *Sports Medicine* 49 (Suppl 2): 115-24. https://doi.org/10.1007/s40279-019-01162-1.

Montain, S.J., and E.F. Coyle. 1992. "Influence of Graded Dehydration on Hyperthermia and Cardiovascular Drift During Exercise." *Journal of Applied Physiology* 73 (4): 1340-50. https://doi.org/10.1152/jappl.1992.73.4.1340.

Sawka, M.N., L.M. Burke, E.R. Eichner, R.J. Maughan, S.J. Montain, and N.S. Stachenfeld. 2007. "American College of Sports Medicine Position Stand: Exercise and Fluid Replacement." *Medicine and Science in Sports and Exercise* 39 (2): 377-90. https:/doi.org/10.1249/mss.0b013e31802ca597.

CHAPTER 4

Academy of Nutrition and Dietetics. 2019. "Healthy Weight During Pregnancy." Last modified August 10, 2020. www.eatright.org/health/pregnancy/prenatal-nutrition/healthy-weight-during-pregnancy.

Academy of Nutrition and Dietetics. 2022. "Nursing Your Baby—What You Eat and Drink Matters." Last modified July 25, 2023. www.eatright.org/health/pregnancy/breastfeeding-and-formula/nursing-your-baby-what-you-eat-and-drink-matters.

Bonjour, J.P. 2011. "Protein Intake and Bone Health." *International Journal for Vitamin and Nutrition Research* 81 (23): 134-42. https://doi.org/10.1024/0300-9831/a000063.

Holtzman, B., and K.E. Ackerman. 2021. "Recommendations and Nutritional Considerations for Female Athletes: Health and Performance." *Sports Medicine* 51 (Suppl 1): 43-57. https://doi.org/10.1007/s40279-021-01508-8.

Horvitz West, E., L. Hark, and D. Deen. 2014. "Nutrition in Pregnancy and Lactation." In *Medical Nutrition and Disease: A Case-Based Approach*, 5th ed., edited by L. Hark, D. Deen, and G. Morrison, 111-45. Chichester, West Sussex, United Kingdom: John Wiley and Sons, Ltd.

Mishra, N., V.N. Mishra, and Devanshi. 2011. "Exercise Beyond Menopause: Dos and Don'ts." *Journal of Mid-Life Health* 2 (2): 51-56. https://doi.org/10.4103/0976-7800.92524.

Mountjoy, M., J.K. Sundgot-Borgen, L.M. Burke, K.E. Ackerman, C. Blauwet, N. Constantini, C. Lebrun et al. 2018. "IOC Consensus Statement on Relative Energy Deficiency in Sport (RED-S): 2018 Update." *British Journal of Sports Medicine* 52 (11): 687-97. https://doi.org/10.1136/bjsports-2018-099193.

Rosen, H.N. 2023. "Patient Education: Calcium and Vitamin D for Bone Health (Beyond the Basics)." Last modified June 12, 2023. www.uptodate.com/contents/calcium-and-vitamin-d-for-bone-health-beyond-the-basics.

Tomiyama, A.J., T. Mann, D. Vinas, J.M. Hunger, J. Dejager, and S.E. Taylor. 2010. "Low Calorie Dieting Increases Cortisol." *Psychosomatic Medicine* 72 (4): 357-64. https://doi.org/10.1097/PSY.0b013e3181d9523c.

Villacis, D., A. Yi, R. Jahn, C.J. Kephart, T. Charlton, S.C. Gamradt, R. Romano, J.E. Tibone, and G.F.R. Hatch, III. 2014. "Prevalence of Abnormal Vitamin D Levels Among Division I NCAA Athletes." *Sports Health* 6 (4): 340-47. https://doi.org/10.1177/1941738114524517.

Yan, H., W. Yang, F. Zhou, X. Li, Q. Pan, Z. Shen, G. Han et al. 2019. "Estrogen Improves Insulin Sensitivity and Suppresses Gluconeogenesis via the Transcription Factor Foxo1." *Diabetes* 68 (2): 291-304. https://doi.org/10.2337/db18-0638.

CHAPTER 5

Chouraqui, J.P. 2022. "Dietary Approaches to Iron Deficiency Prevention in Childhood—A Critical Public Health Issue." *Nutrients* 14 (8): 1604. https://doi.org/10.3390/nu14081604.

Medawar, E., S. Huhn, A. Villringer, and A.V. Witte. 2019. "The Effects of Plant-Based Diets on the Body and the Brain: A Systematic Review." *Translational Psychiatry* 9, 226. https://doi.org/10.1038/s41398-019-0552-0.

Monsen, E.R. 1988. "Iron Nutrition and Absorption: Dietary Factors Which Impact Iron Bioavailability." *Journal of the American Dietetic Association* 88 (7): 786-90.

National Institutes of Health. 2023. "Iron: Fact Sheet for Consumers." Last modified August 17, 2023. https://ods.od.nih.gov/factsheets/Iron-Consumer/.

Rakhra, G., D. Masih, A. Vats, S.K. Verma, V.K. Singh, V. Kirar, and S.N. Singh. 2021. "Effect of Endurance Training on Copper, Zinc, Iron and Magnesium Status." *Jour-

nal of Sports Medicine and Physical Fitness 61 (9): 1273-80. https://doi.org/10.23736/S0022-4707.21.11647-0.

Shaw, K., G.A. Zello, C. Rodgers, T. Warkentin, A. Baerwald. and P. Chilibeck. 2022. "Benefits of a Plant-Based Diet and Considerations for the Athlete." *European Journal of Applied Physiology* 122:1163-78. https://doi.org/10.1007/s00421-022-04902-w.

Tso, R., and C.G. Forde. 2021. "Unintended Consequences: Nutritional Impact and Potential Pitfalls of Switching from Animal- to Plant-Based Foods." *Nutrients* 13 (8): 2527. https://doi.org/10.3390/nu13082527.

CHAPTER 6

Canavan, C., J. West, and T. Card. 2014. "The Epidemiology of Irritable Bowel Syndrome." *Clinical Epidemiology* 6:71-80. https://doi.org/10.2147/CLEP.S40245.

Crowe, S.E. 2019. "Food Allergy vs Food Intolerance in Patients With Irritable Bowel Syndrome." *Gastroenterology and Hepatology* 15 (1): 38-40.

de Oliveira, E.P., R.C. Burini, and A. Jeukendrup. 2014. "Gastrointestinal Complaints During Exercise: Prevalence, Etiology, and Nutritional Recommendations." *Sports Medicine* 44 (Suppl 1): S79-85. https://doi.org/10.1007/s40279-014-0153-2.

Roszkowska, A., M. Pawlicka, A. Mroczek, K. Bałabuszek, and B. Nieradko-Iwanicka. 2019. "Non-Celiac Gluten Sensitivity: A Review." *Medicina* 55 (6): 222. https://doi.org/10.3390/medicina55060222.

U.S. Food and Drug Administration. 2023. "Food Allergies." Last modified April 12, 2024. www.fda.gov/food/food-labeling-nutrition/food-allergies.

Wiffin, M., L. Smith, J. Antonio, J. Johnstone, L. Beasley, and J. Roberts. 2019. "Effect of a Short-Term Low Fermentable Oligiosaccharide, Disaccharide, Monosaccharide and Polyol (FODMAP) Diet on Exercise-Related Gastrointestinal Symptoms." *Journal of the International Society of Sports Nutrition* 16 (1): 1. https://doi.org/10.1186/s12970-019-0268-9.

CHAPTER 7

Snijders, T., J. Trommelen, I.W.K. Kouw, A.M. Holwerda, L.B. Verdijk, and L.J.C. van Loon. 2019. "The Impact of Pre-Sleep Protein Ingestion on the Skeletal Muscle Adaptive Response to Exercise in Humans: An Update." *Frontiers in Nutrition* 6, 17. https://doi.org/10.3389/fnut.2019.00017.

CHAPTER 8

Bergström, J., L. Hermansen, E. Hultman, and B. Saltin. 1967. "Diet, Muscle Glycogen and Physical Performance." *Acta Physiologica Scandinavica* 71 (2): 140-50. https://doi.org/10.1111/j.1748-1716.1967.tb03720.x.

FISA, the World Rowing Federation. 2002. "Basic Rowing Physiology." In *The FISA Coaching Development Programme: Handbook—Level II*, edited by T.S. Nilsen, T. Daigneault, and M. Smith, 24-37. Lausanne, Switzerland: FISA - The International Rowing Federation. https://worldrowing.com/wp-content/uploads/2020/12/Level2%EA%9E%89Chapter2%EA%9E%89BasicRowingPhysiology_English.pdf.

Kelly, D.J., A. Nepotiuk, and L.E. Brown. 2021. "Rowing Performance After Dehydration: An Unexpected Effect of Method." *SportRχiv*. https://doi.org/10.31236/osf.io/pv9dw.

Kim, J., and E.K. Kim. 2020. "Nutritional Strategies to Optimize Performance and Recovery in Rowing Athletes." *Nutrients* 12 (6): 1685. https://doi.org/10.3390/nu12061685.

Oliver, B. 2019. "How Ron Hill Ate His Way Into Marathon Running History." Inside the Games. Last modified September 22, 2019. www.insidethegames.biz/articles/1085027/ron-hill-marathon-innovator-big-read.

Sherman, W.M., D.L. Costill, W.J. Fink, and J.M. Miller. 1981. "Effect of Exercise-Diet Manipulation on Muscle Glycogen and its Subsequent Utilization During Performance." *International Journal of Sports Medicine* 2 (2): 114-18. https://doi.org/10.1055/s-2008-1034594.

CHAPTER 9

Bergström, J., L. Hermansen, E. Hultman, and B. Saltin. 1967. "Diet, Muscle Glycogen and Physical Performance." *Acta Physiologica Scandinavica* 71 (2): 140-50. https://doi.org/10.1111/j.1748-1716.1967.tb03720.x.

de Oliveira, E.P., R.C. Burini, and A. Jeukendrup. 2014. "Gastrointestinal Complaints During Exercise: Prevalence, Etiology, and Nutritional Recommendations." *Sports Medicine* 44 (Suppl 1): S79-85. https://doi.org/10.1007/s40279-014-0153-2.

Glace, B., C. Murphy, and M. McHugh. 2002. "Food and Fluid Intake and Disturbances in Gastrointestinal and Mental Function During an Ultramarathon." *International Journal of Sport Nutrition and Exercise Metabolism* 12 (4): 414-27. https://doi.org/10.1123/ijsnem.12.4.414.

Jeukendrup, A.E. 2010. "Carbohydrate and Exercise Performance: The Role of Multiple Transportable Carbohydrates." *Current Opinion in Clinical Nutrition and Metabolic Care* 13 (4): 452-57. https://doi.org/10.1097/MCO.0b013e328339de9f.

Shirreffs, S.M., and M.N. Sawka. 2011. "Fluid and Electrolyte Needs for Training, Competition, and Recovery." *Journal of Sports Sciences* 29 (Suppl 1): S39-46. https://doi.org/10.1080/02640414.2011.614269.

Tiller, N.B., J.D. Roberts, L. Beasley, S. Chapman, J.M. Pinto, L. Smith, M. Wiffin et al. 2019. "International Society of Sports Nutrition Position Stand: Nutritional Considerations for Single-Stage Ultra-Marathon Training and Racing." *Journal of the International Society of Sport Nutrition* 16 (1): 50. https://doi.org/10.1186/s12970-019-0312-9.

CHAPTER 10

Aragon, A.A., and B.J. Schoenfeld. 2013. "Nutrient Timing Revisited: Is There a Post-Exercise Anabolic Window?" *Journal of the International Society of Sports Nutrition* 10 (1): 5. https://doi.org/10.1186/1550-2783-10-5.

Jentjens, R., and A. Jeukendrup. 2003. "Determinants of Post-Exercise Glycogen Synthesis During Short-Term Recovery." *Sports Medicine* 33:117-44. https://doi.org/10.2165/00007256-200333020-00004.

Samuels, C., and L. James. 2014. "Sleep as a Recovery Tool for Athletes." *British Journal of Sports Medicine* (blog). Last modified November 17, 2014. http://blogs.bmj.com/bjsm/2014/11/17/6066/.

Vella, L.D., and D. Cameron-Smith. 2010. "Alcohol, Athletic Performance and Recovery." *Nutrients* 2 (8): 781-89. https://doi.org/10.3390/nu2080781.

USDA Food Data Central. Food Search. https://fdc.nal.usda.gov/fdc-app.html#/food-search?query=&type=Foundation. Accessed: August 27, 2024.

INDEX

ABOUT THE AUTHOR

Kylee Van Horn, RDN, is a registered dietitian nutritionist and founder of Fly-nutrition LLC, a virtual sports nutrition private practice that exclusively serves the endurance athlete population. With a mission of separating facts from fads, Van Horn provides practical guidance for endurance athletes to direct them to a sustainable approach to fueling their activities for long-term health and performance.

Van Horn writes a monthly nutrition column published in *Outside Run Magazine* and has written for *FasterSkier* and *Gnarly Sports Nutrition*. She is quoted frequently in articles for *Outside Magazine* and speaks regularly to athletes and professionals on topics related to endurance sports nutrition for running, skiing, climbing, triathlon, obstacle course racing, and mountaineering. She is the cohost of the podcast *Your Diet Sucks*, which seeks to provide thoughtful conversations—backed by science—around controversial topics in the diet and fitness space. She has also been featured on numerous podcasts, including *The Running Explained Podcast*, *The Strength Running Podcast*, *Consummate Athlete*, *Bodies in Motion*, and *Off the Couch*.

A competitive endurance athlete since the age of 10, Van Horn is certified as a USATF Level 1 Running Coach and has worked in endurance event production since 2009 (for World Triathlon and local races). She studied veterinary medicine and biology at the University of Richmond, where she ran Division I cross country and track and field and graduated with her BA degree in 2008. She received her BS degree in human nutrition from Metropolitan State University of Denver in 2013 and completed her dietetic internship at the University of Northern Colorado in 2018. When she's not talking about nutrition, Van Horn is on her home trails near Aspen, Colorado, with her ultra-endurance athlete husband, Sean, and their three Australian shepherds.

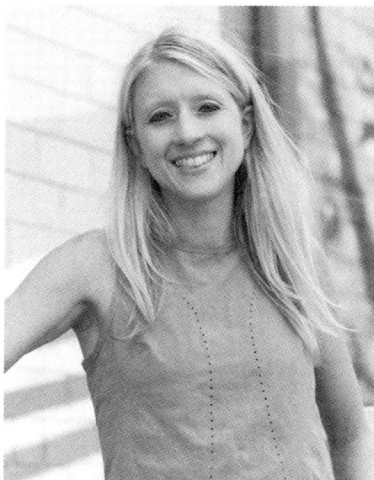